REV Med

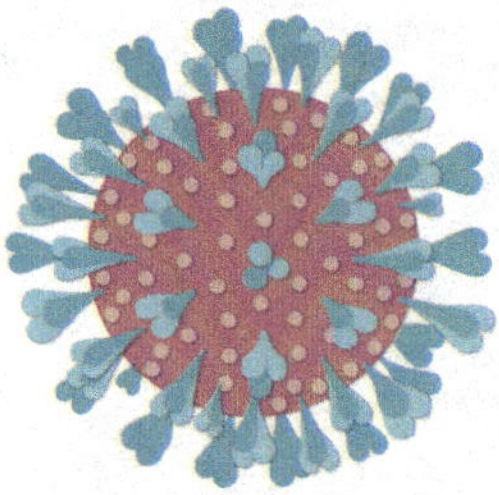

COVID-19

THE REASON WHY THE EARTH STOOD STILL IN 2020

An illustrated guide to understanding the virus: **SARS-CoV-2**

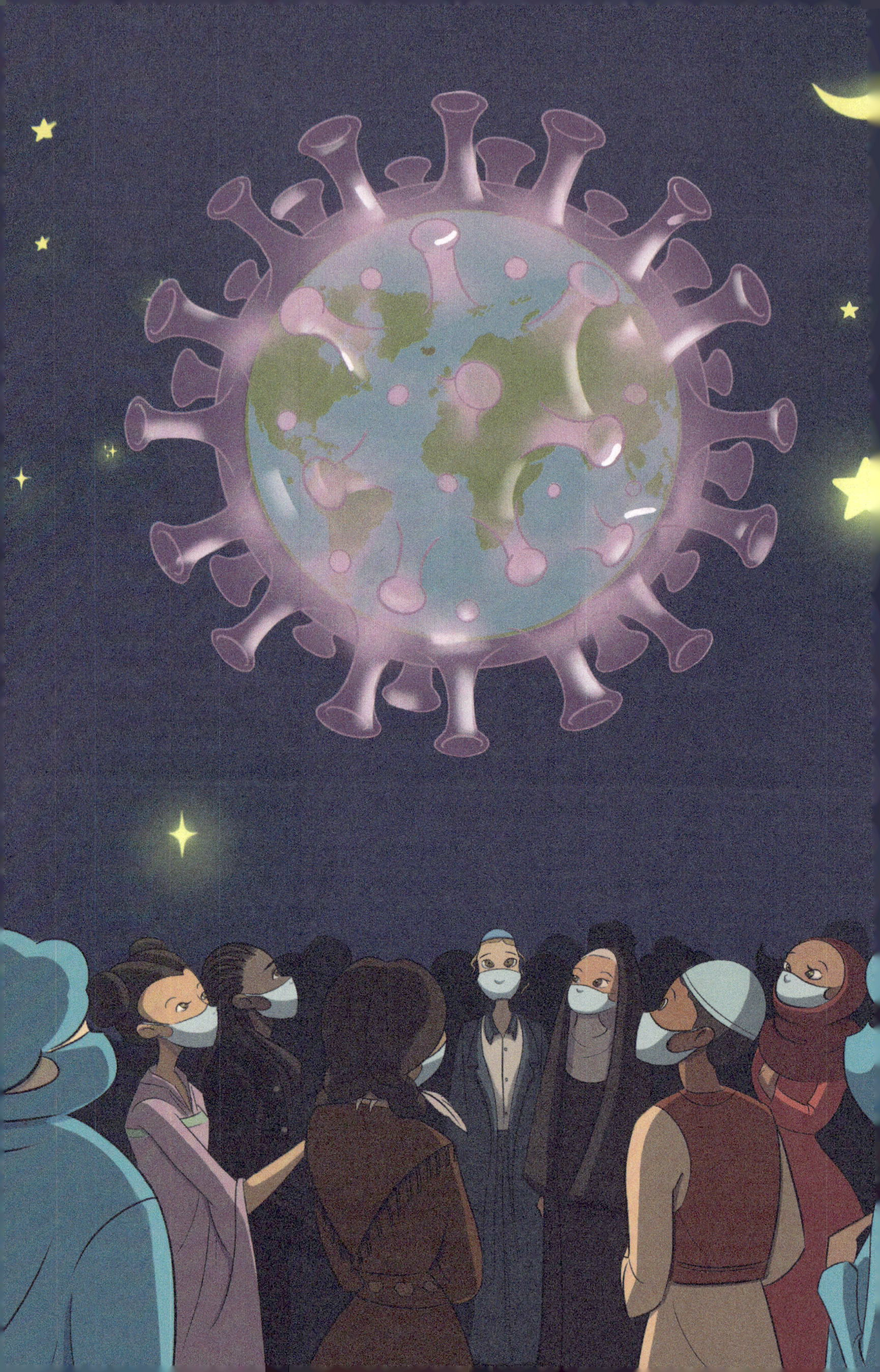

REV Med

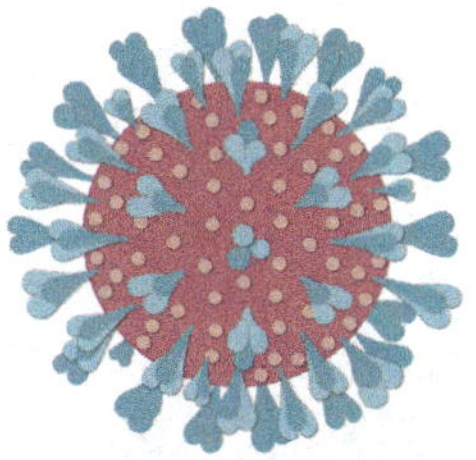

FIRST EDITION

COVID-19

THE REASON WHY THE EARTH STOOD STILL IN 2020

An illustrated guide to understanding the virus: **SARS-CoV-2**

Syed M. Rizvi
LEAD EDUCATOR
@rev.med
REV MED | ONLINE MEDICAL EDUCATION PLATFORM
NEW YORK, US

Pippasha Khan
DENTAL SURGEON
@drpippa.k
KING'S COLLEGE
LONDON, UK

Rebecca Caruana
FACULTY
MEDICINE AND SURGERY
UNIVERSITY OF MALTA
MSIDA, MALTA

Daniel Hrbolic
SPEECH LANGUAGE PATHOLOGY
@thestudyingslp
LA TROBE UNIVERSITY
MELBOURNE, AU

First Printing, 2022

Library of Congress Control Number: 2020925714

ISBN: 978-0-578-83212-8

For rights and permissions, please contact:

REV MED

New York, NY

covid19ebook@gmail.com

www.covid19ebook.org

@REV.MED

DISCLAIMER

The authors of **COVID-19: The Reason Why the Earth Stood Still in 2020** have made every effort to provide information that is accurate and complete as of the date of publication. However, in view of the rapid changes occurring in medical science, COVID-19 prevention, policy, incoming research, and the possibility of human error, this text may contain technical inaccuracies, typographical, or other errors. Readers are thus advised to check all current and relevant information via cdc.gov, who.int, or local health authorities.

The contents of this book, such as, text, links, images, and other materials created by or obtained for **COVID-19: The Reason Why the Earth Stood Still in 2020**, and other materials found on the **COVID-19: The Reason Why the Earth Stood Still in 2020** web platforms are for informational and educational purposes only.

This book is not engaged in rendering medical and current historical advice or professional services. Furthermore, the content is not intended to be a substitute for medical advice, diagnosis, or treatment. Members of the general public reading this book are advised to always seek advice from a physician or other qualified health provider regarding personal medical care. If you have, or suspect that you may have, a health problem, consult your healthcare provider immediately.

CONTRIBUTING AUTHORS AND ADVISORY BOARD

Dr. Uzma Syed, DO

INFECTIOUS DISEASE SPECIALIST
COVID-19 TASK FORCE CHAIR

@uzmasworld

GOOD SAMARITAN HOSPITAL MEDICAL CENTER
SOUTH SHORE INFECTIOUS DISEASES
BAY SHORE, NY, US

Dr. Arunabh Talwar, MD

ADV. LUNG DISEASE SPECIALIST
PULMONOLOGIST AND EDUCATOR

@rev.med

DONALD & BARBARA ZUCKER SCHOOL OF MEDICINE AT HOFSTRA/NORTHWELL
HEMPSTEAD, NY, US

Dr. Ailia Rizvi, DO

CARDIOVASCULAR DISEASE
CARDIOLOGIST AND EDUCATOR

@rev.med

ARNOT OGDEN MEDICAL CENTER
ELMIRA, NY, US

Mesha Mustafa, BScN, RN

ORTHOPEDIC SURGERY
REGISTERED NURSE

OVERLAKE HOSPITAL MEDICAL CENTER
BELLEVUE, WA, US

Joao Costa

MEDICAL EDUCATOR
COFOUNDER OF KENHUB

@kenhub_official

KENHUB
GERMANY
WWW.KENHUB.COM

Dr. Julie Groveman, PsyD

CLINICAL PSYCHOLOGY
LICENSED PSYCHOLOGIST

@askdoctorjulie

PRIVATE PRACTICE
NEW YORK, NY, US
WWW.ASKDOCJULIE.COM

Barbara Olas, RN

CARDIOLOGY
REGISTERED NURSE

@yournursingeducator

ONTARIO, CANADA

Laura Jane Jones

DIGITAL ILLUSTRATOR

@laurajaneillustrations

HELLO HAPPEE
ITALY
WWW.HELLOHAPPEE.COM

EDITORIAL ASSISTANCE

Moira Cross

PROOFREADER, TRANSLATOR & TRANSCRIBER

/moiracrossproofreader

MALTA

Andy Meaden

GRAPHIC DESIGNER
BOOK COMPILATION

www.meadencreative.com

MEADEN CREATIVE | GRAPHIC DESIGN
LONDON, UK

DEDICATION

To all the healthcare workers on the frontlines and caregivers at home, we dedicate this book to you, for the sacrifices you make each and every day, and especially, during such times as the COVID-19 pandemic. Your commitment, dedication, and courage deserve an applause. We extend our deepest admiration and gratitude to you for saving so many lives and leaving an indelible mark on the hearts of many.

We cannot say or do much to express how thankful we are. However, do always know that, each time you scrub in, put on your uniform, and take on the virus, we are able to sleep better at night, simply knowing that there are people like you who exist in this world.

WE WOULD LIKE TO SAY...

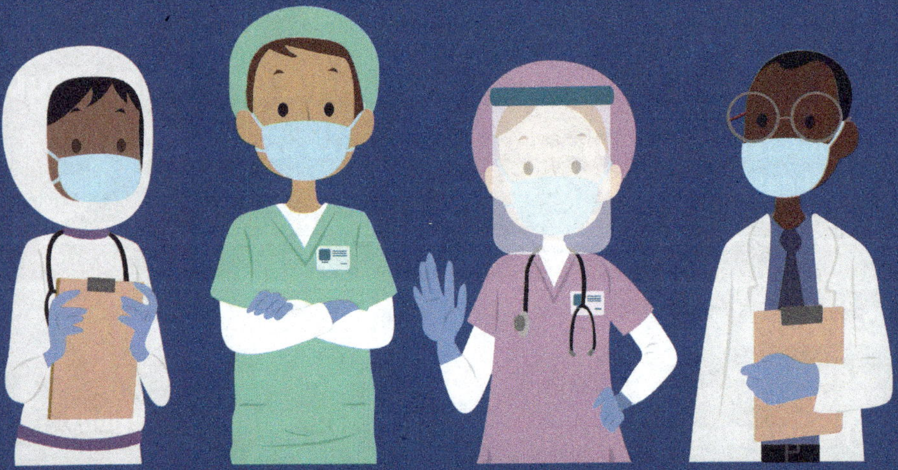

Shnorhakalut'yun Salamat **Misaotra** Tack **Rahmat**
Ευχαριστώ 감사합니다 Grazzi شكرا لك Teşekkürler **Dhanyabaad**
Danke **Grazie** ขอบคุณ **Kám-siā** Спасибо **Sipas dikim** Köszönöm
Благодаря Amesegnalaw **Gracias** Asante **çox sağ olun** Dhanyavadalu
Mulțumesc धन्यवाद **Danke** Ngiyabonga
Hvala **Mahadsanid** Dhonobad **ābhāra**

Thank you.

Děkuji Dank u شكريه **Dhanwaad** Stutiyi
Deu borem korum Obrigado **Manana**
Kiitos 谢谢你 Nandri **Arkun** Terima kasih **Cè-zù tin-ba-deh** Meharbani
A ni kié Urakoze **Tak** תודה **Dziękuję** سپاسگزارم **Zikomo** Shukriya
Ke a leboga Dziakuj **Дякую** **Na gode** **Kan sia** Murakoze
Mèsi **Nandi** Merci ありがとうございます Cảm ơn

PREFACE

In 2020, healthcare workers, first responders, security personnel, and maintenance staff were standing fearlessly on the frontlines taking on COVID-19. This dedication motivated us to do our part and provide a reliable source to educate the general public.

We realized quickly that this disease was not only spreading into the cities or towns we live in, but was reaching a global scale. Therefore, our response in writing this book had to be an international effort. We thus assembled our team of medical experts and students from countries across the world, all united to offer a well-versed and illustrated overview of the COVID-19 pandemic.

Not only did we have family and friends who were affected by the virus, SARS-CoV-2, but we saw our colleagues work tirelessly around the clock. These heroes struggled hard to prevent further cases and care for those falling ill. In times like this, we become overwhelmed, and ask such questions as: "What is this virus?" or "When will life be normal again?" This book aims to not only answer these questions, but also provide a reliable source of information that is concise and easy to understand.

Rest assured that the contents of this book were examined by our advisory board, consisting of a COVID-19 task force chair, medical professors, and specialty experts. The information found throughout this book is in parallel and sourced from reliable organizations, such as, the World Health Organization (WHO), the Centers for Disease Control and Prevention (CDC), and local health authorities.

This project did come with its challenges. With the constant change of medical prognosis, care, and advice, it was a race against time for us to get the content out to the public. We set aside countless hours, working day and night for several months. This project was not funded or backed by grants; instead, we committed our time and energy for one sole purpose: the betterment of humanity amidst a pandemic.

Lastly, as we move on to our new reality, life post-pandemic, and are released from our confines, we must take a look at how our physical and mental health has changed. Going forward, we will appreciate the earth because, while we were caged, the earth continued its life and remained beautiful, and we stood still in fear. When we are back, let us remember that we are only its guests, and not its masters.

We hope you find value in this book, and we wish you good health, safety, and continued love for the earth and humanity,

Syed M. Rizvi — NEW YORK

Pippasha Khan — LONDON

Daniel Hrbolic — MELBOURNE

Rebecca Caruana — MALTA

TIMELINE

Dec 31, 2019

China notifies the world!

Chinese authorities notified the world about pneumonia cases in Wuhan city, Hubei province, China, with an unknown cause and spreading through their communities.

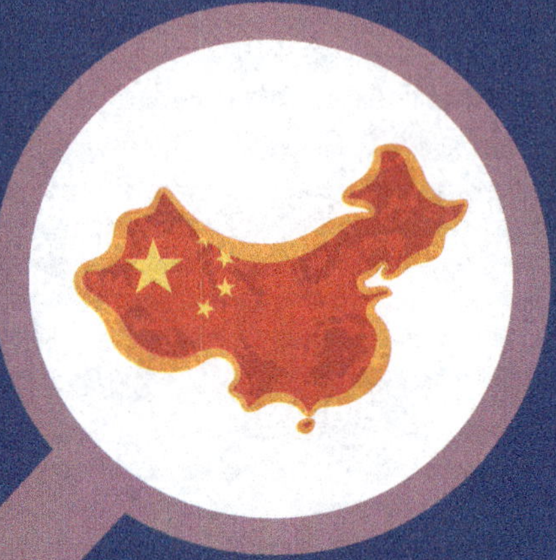

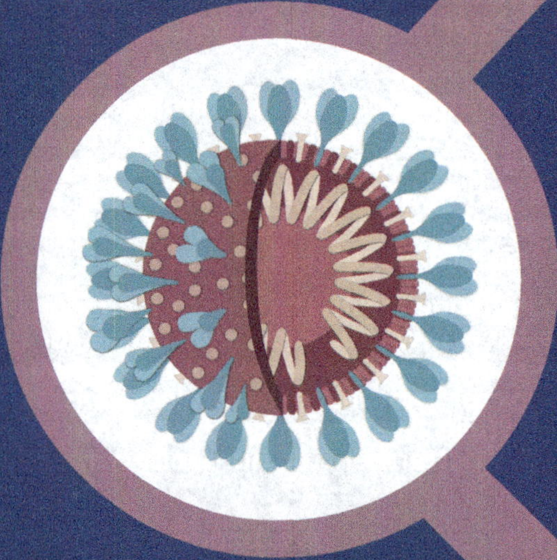

Jan 12, 2020

China shares more information

Authorities publicly share the genetic sequence of COVID-19.

Feb 16-24, 2020

WHO-China Joint Mission

Experts from Canada, Germany, Japan, Nigeria, Republic of Korea, Russia, Singapore, and the US (CDC, NIH) were invited to Beijing and Wuhan. They spoke with health officials, scientists, and health workers.

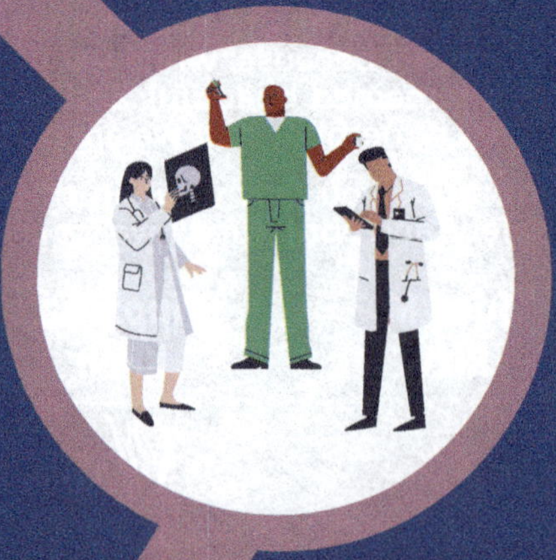

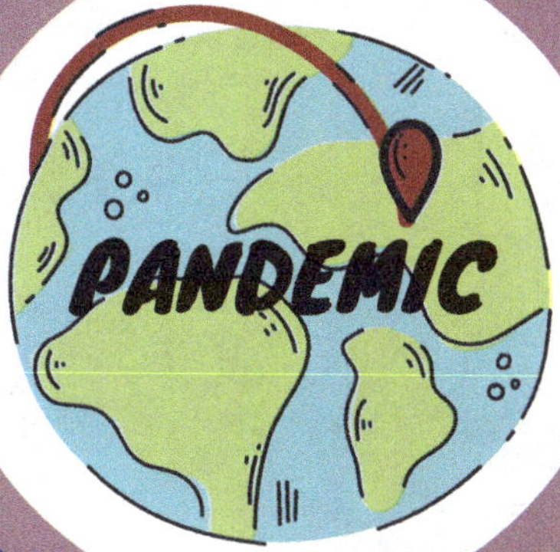

Mar 11, 2020

Declared a Pandemic

After deeply concerned by the alarming levels of spread, severity, and inaction, the World Health Organization (WHO) declared that the disease COVID-19 was to be characterized as a pandemic.

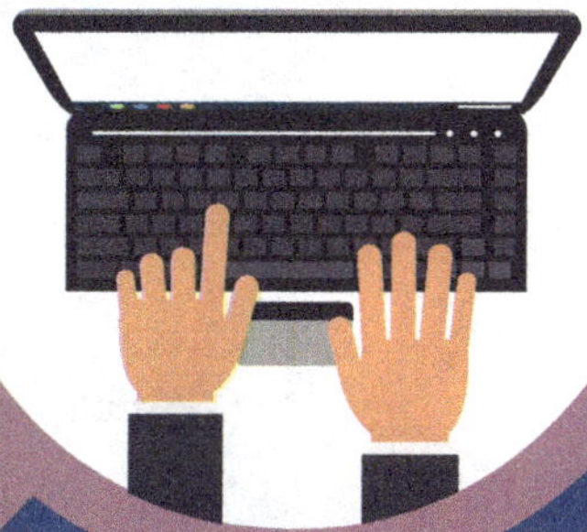

Mar 30, 2020

United Nations Global Call

UN issues a global call and open brief to creatives in order to help stop the spread of COVID-19.

NOW

Our Team assembles to write a COVID-19 guide book!

We responded by creating a task force of authors and medical experts to write behind the front1lines of the pandemic. We now introduce the illustrated guide to understanding SARS-CoV-2.

TABLE OF CONTENTS

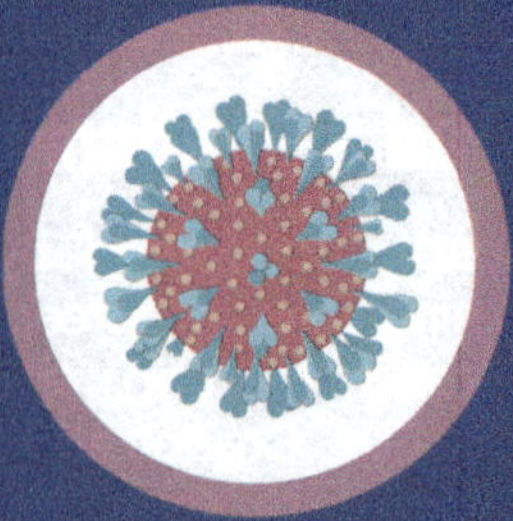

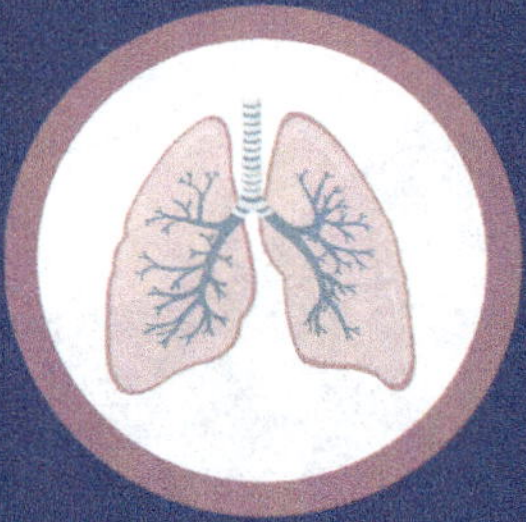

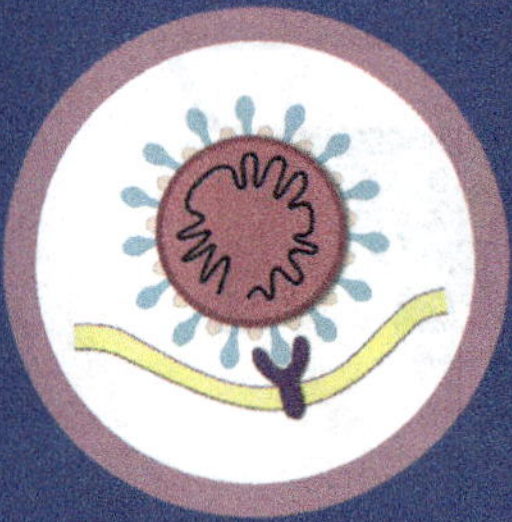

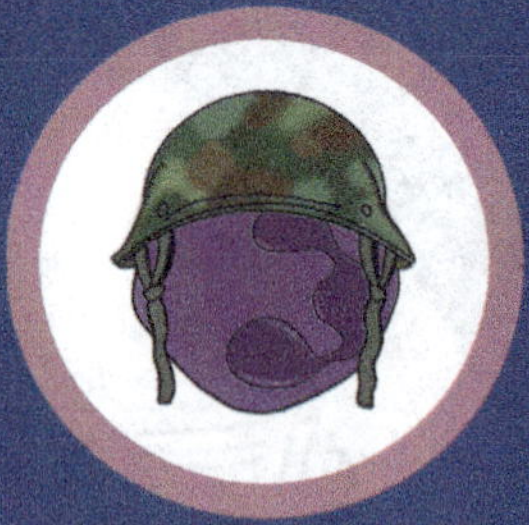

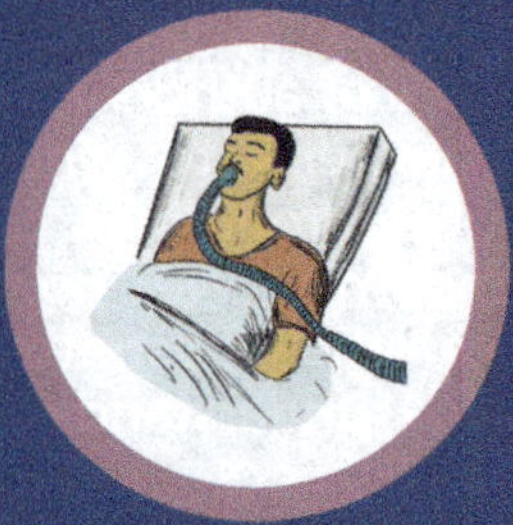

TABLE OF CONTENTS

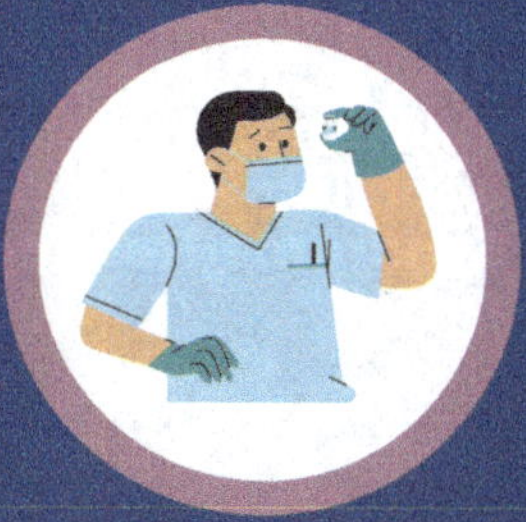

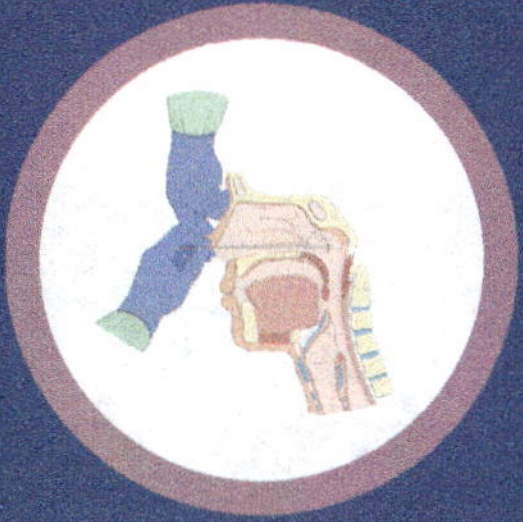

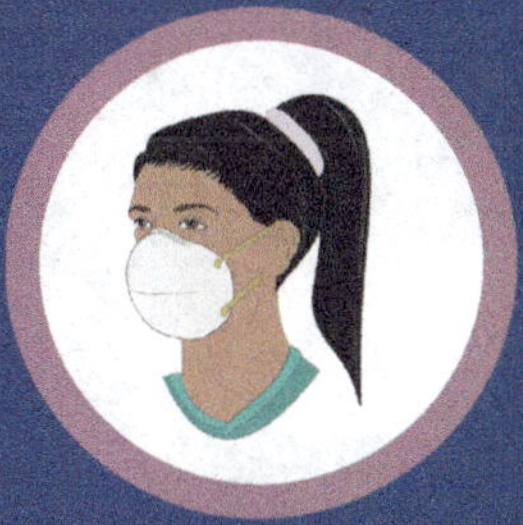

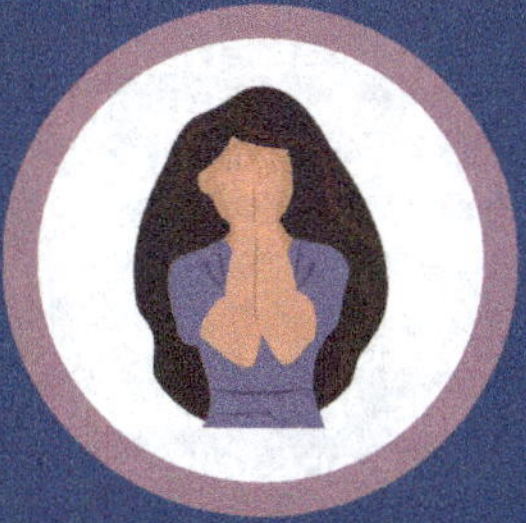

SUMMARY

In December 2019, Chinese health authorities notified the world that a virus was spreading through their communities. In the following months, it spread to other countries, with cases doubling within days. The virus is the **'Severe Acute Respiratory Syndrome-Related Coronavirus 2'**.

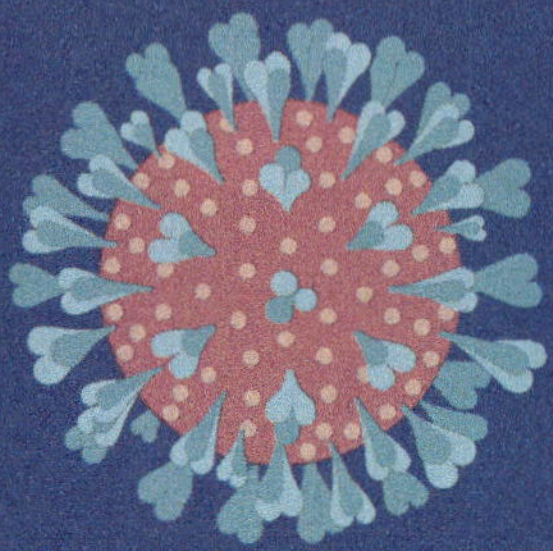

We'll call it

SARS-CoV-2

In February 2020, the World Health Organization announced an official name for the disease – COVID-19.

Virus 2019

COVID-19

Corona Disease

CORONAVIRUS

Coronaviruses are a large family of viruses that cause mild to moderate upper-respiratory tract illnesses in humans. In the past two decades, there have been serious and fatal coronaviruses, such as, SARS-CoV, which emerged in November 2002, causing the disease SARS and MERS-CoV in September 2012, eventually causing MERS. The third novel coronavirus to emerge in this century is SARS-CoV-2, causing COVID-19, which everyone simply calls 'coronavirus'. How does it actually infect a human, what happens when it infects, and what should we all do?

1 What is a Virus?

- What does a Virus look like?
- Origin of Viruses
- How does a Virus multiply?

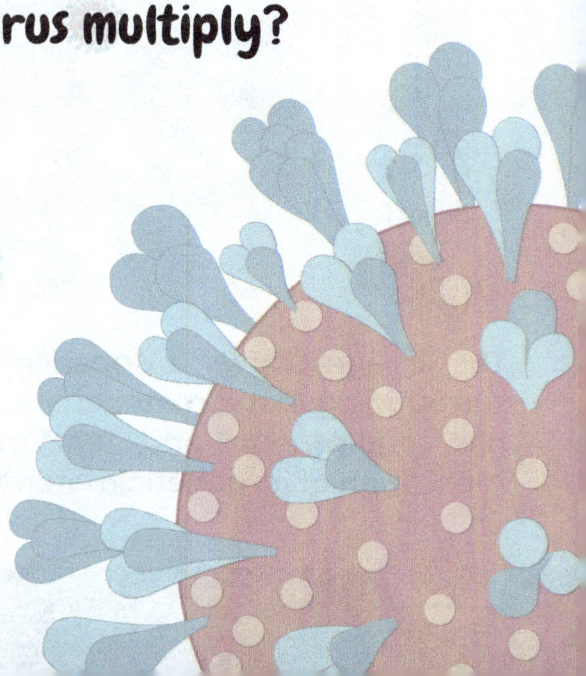

What is a Virus?

For many years, scientists have debated over what a virus actually is. Are viruses living or non-living?

Most people define life by particular qualities, such as, being able to replicate, or being bound by the aspects of birth and death. Interestingly, viruses themselves cannot replicate or survive on their own, but they can survive by entering living cells, thus affecting the behavior of their 'hosts'.

What does a Virus look like?

Viruses come in different shapes, such as, polyhedral, complex, helical, and enveloped. Viruses such as Influenza and HIV, which are enveloped, are surrounded by a membrane that includes proteins that seek out cells to infect.

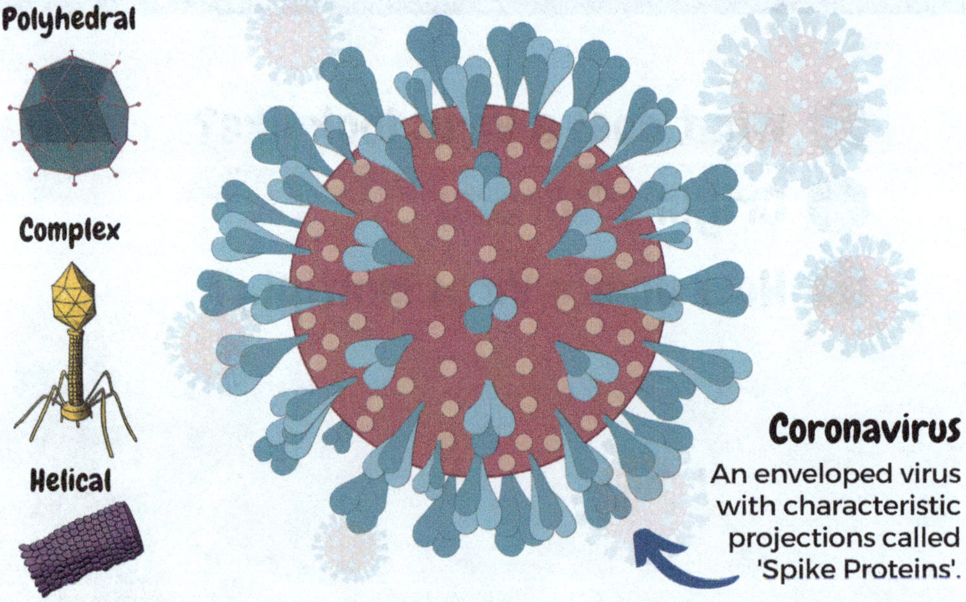

This image shows a spherically enveloped particle which surrounds genetic material and structural proteins. The virus has equipment and enzymes for manipulation and replication of its genetic material.

What is a Virus?

The coronavirus, for example, is an enveloped virus which contains a single strand of positive-sense RNA. It is spherical, with structural proteins, such as, the envelope (E), membrane (M), and genetic material (nucleocapsid-N). The key to the infection pathway of the virus is its pronounced Spike proteins (S), which are embedded in the envelope.

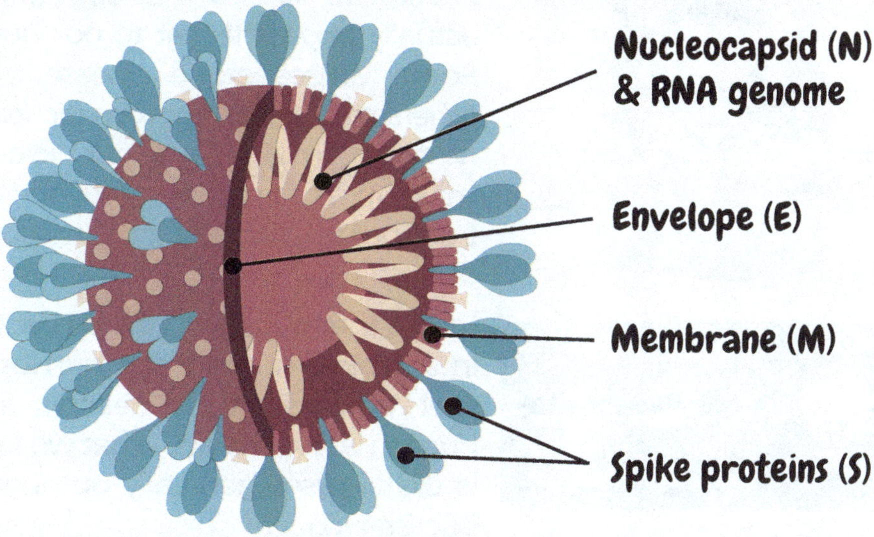

A virus is arguably not even a living thing. It can only make more of itself by entering a living cell and self-replicating.

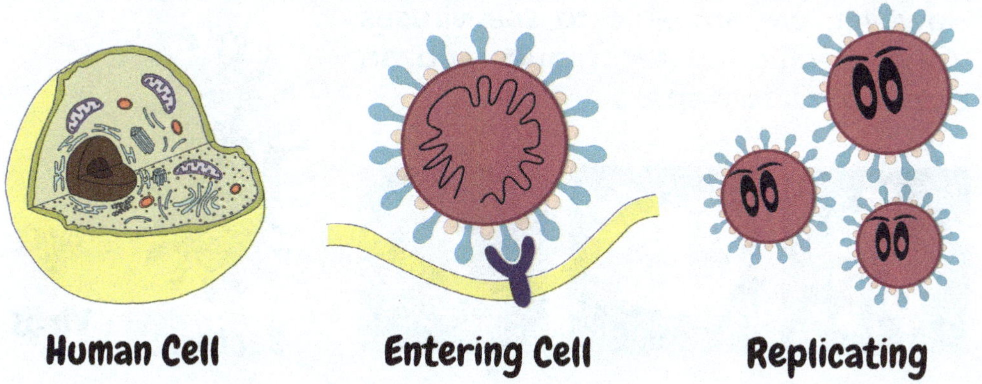

What is a Virus?

Viruses are everywhere, from our surroundings, to the very food we eat. We ingest, inhale, and take in millions of viruses every second.

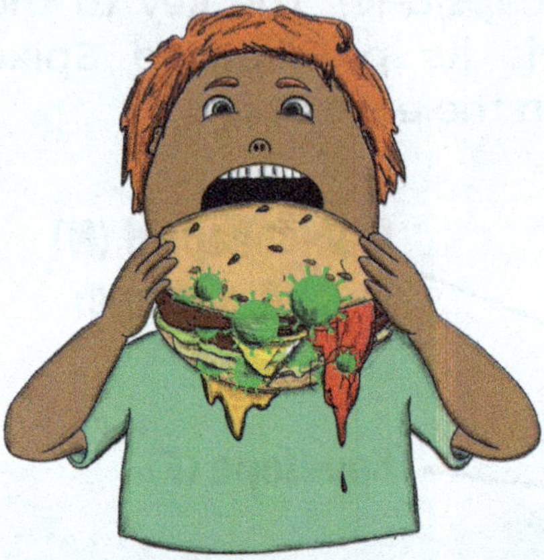

Humans live relatively free of illness, even though the world is filled with viruses. This is because only a small fraction of viruses that surround us actually pose a threat to our bodies. Some viruses cause disease, while others may be asymptomatic (cause no symptoms) because our biological makeup is great at preventing us from being infected, for the most part, at least!

Interestingly there are more viruses than stars in the universe, but only some will infect us!

Unlike the roughly 40 trillion bacteria in a typical human, the number of viral particles in a healthy adult human is not known. What we know is that viruses generally outnumber bacteria 10:1.

Viruses are microscopic, and are so tiny that, even if bacteria had eyes... they would not be able to see them!

However, we are able to see viruses using specific lab techniques and an electron microscope.

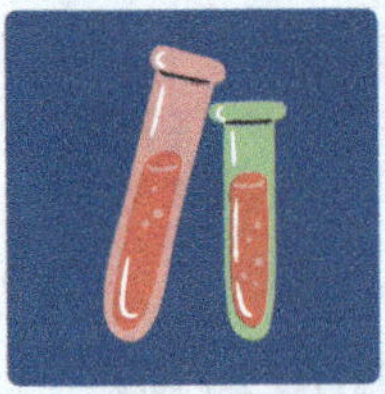

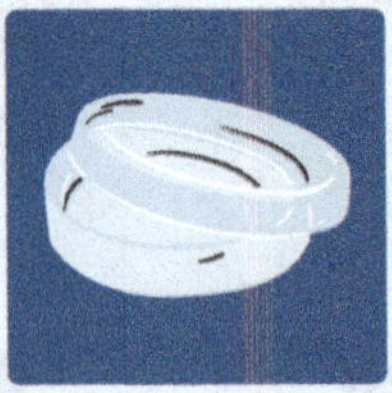

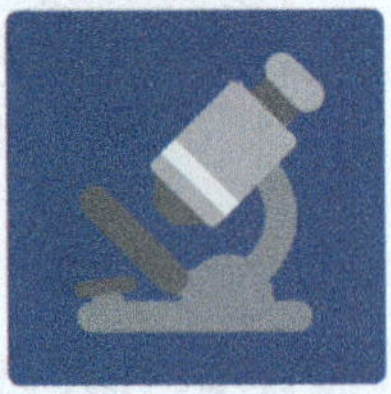

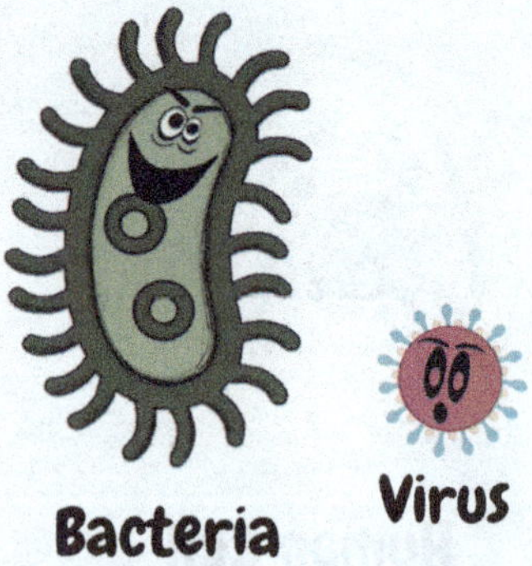

Origin of Viruses

It is difficult to pin down where a virus originates, and studying the ancestry of viruses can be a huge task. This is because viruses have the ability to stick their own genes into the cells they infect. Therefore, figuring out the historical point of which host or organism it first infected can be close to impossible. Viruses do not leave any fossils, and not only do they infect humans, but they can also infect any organism, from bacteria to bats, to people.

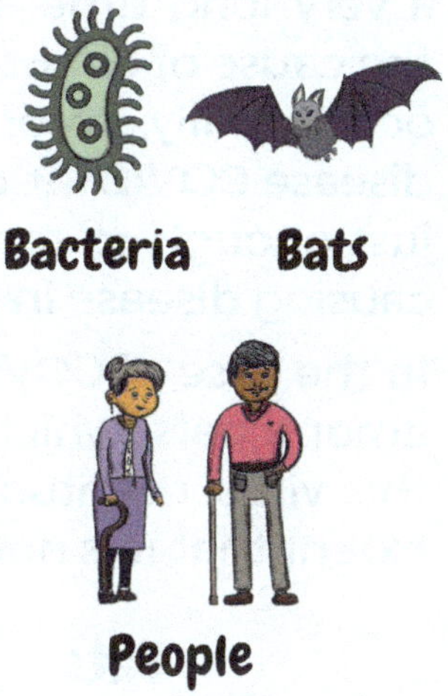

Yet, many scientists believe that viruses began as big bits of cellular DNA and then became independent—or that these viruses came along very early in evolution, and some of their DNA stuck around in the DNA of other cells.

In fact, some scientists even believe that the first human cell (in our existence) was formed from a virus which infected a bacterium billions of years ago and helped form our cell nucleus.

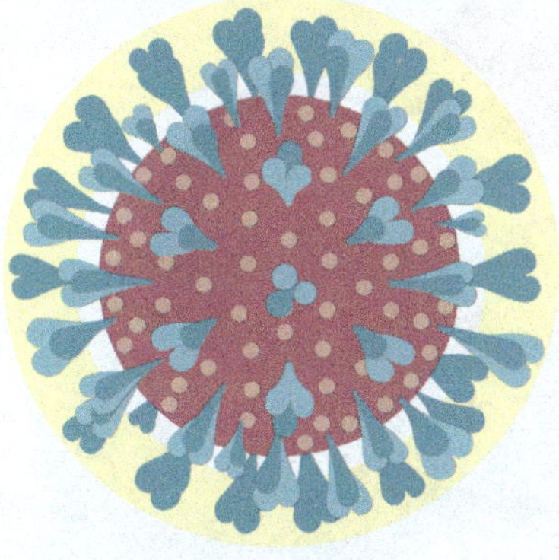

Coronaviruses are not new viruses as some may think. The spikes on the surface of coronaviruses give this virus family its name—corona, which is Latin for 'crown', since any coronavirus would have a crown-like appearance. This appears as a halo surrounding the envelope as seen in electron microscopy.

What is a Virus?

Most coronaviruses have been circulating among humans for a very long time and are typically benign. They are actually the cause of about a quarter of all common cold illnesses. Yet, occasionally, coronaviruses such as SARS-CoV-2, causing the disease COVID-19, circulate in an animal reservoir, and mutate just enough to reach a stage where they start infecting and causing disease in humans.

In the case of COVID-19, researchers detected the coronavirus among bats, which are natural animal reservoirs. They believe the virus eventually mutated, and as of late 2019, to the extent that it is now causing disease in humans.

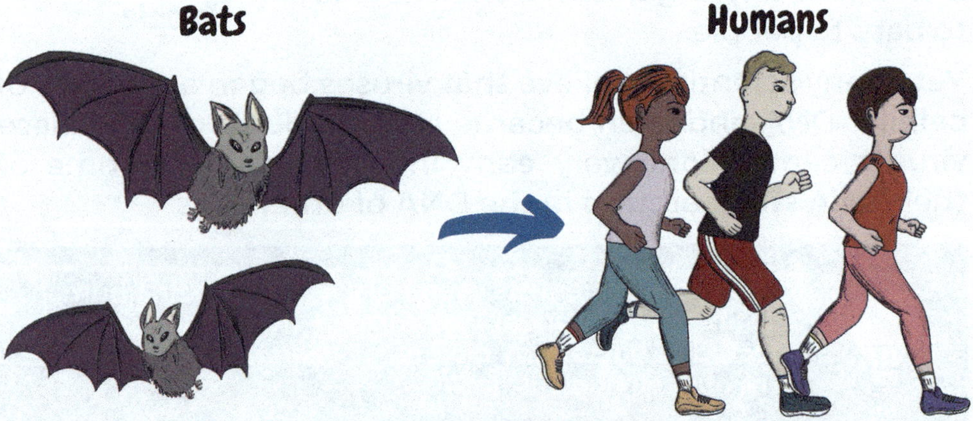

Even though SARS-CoV-2 began from China, it has since traveled throughout the world, infecting millions of people. The virus is able to infect at high rates because it has the ability to replicate and multiply.

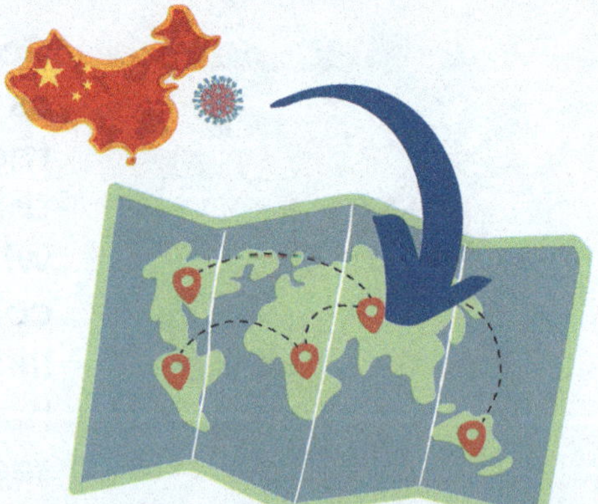

How does a Virus multiply?

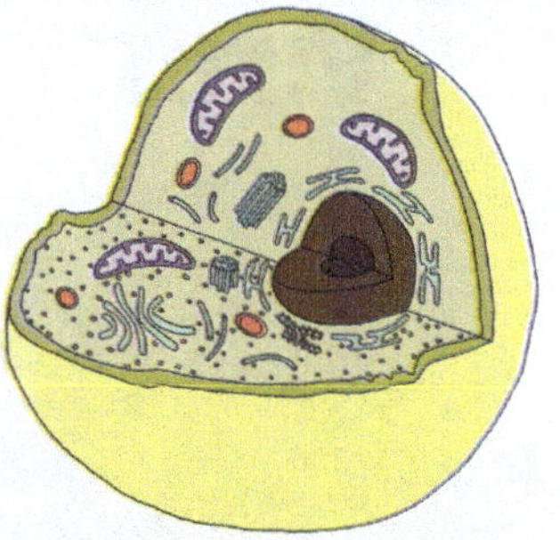

A virus uses its genome with various molecular machinery to replicate itself; however, it cannot do this alone. It must find a host to infect. Our body cells are the perfect home for viruses.

Armed with their genetic material, viruses are able to infect healthy cells, and convert them into mindless virus-producing zombies.

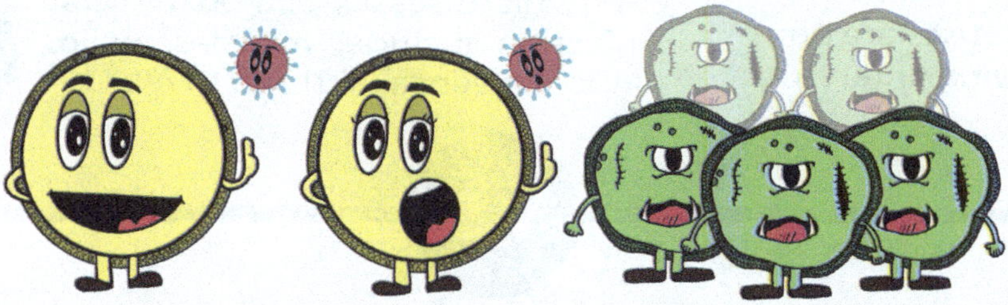

The virus uses its outer protein coat covered in small molecular receptors to bind and join to the membrane of a cell. This is essential for it determines which cell a virus is able to infect. Once joined, the virus uses several complicated biological pathways in order to force the cell to either accept its genetic material, or take in the entire virus.

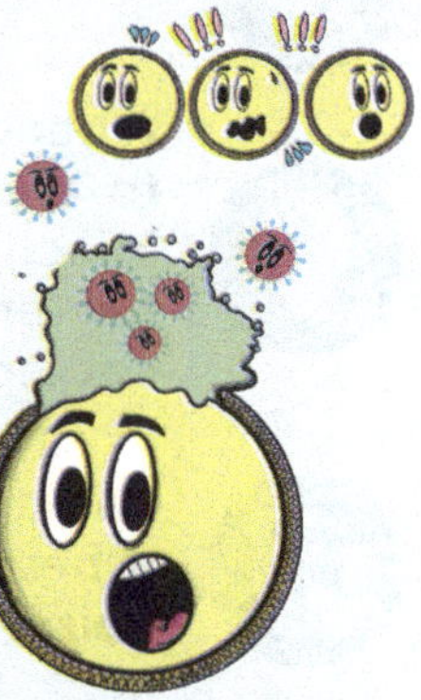

Inside the cell, the virus will begin to use its molecular weapons to overtake the cell's protein manufacturing systems and its DNA replication mechanism.

These viruses then cause tension in the cell, and thus, burst out with the intention of infecting new hosts for the same purpose...

Multiplying the virus.

What is a Virus?

Virus

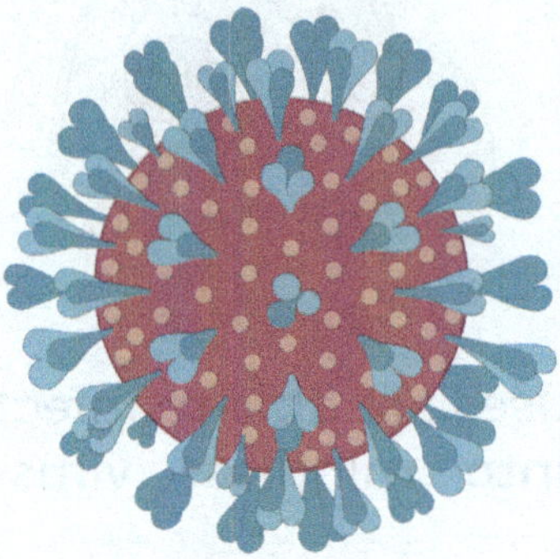

Viruses are non-living organisms

Virion only grow and reproduce inside the host cells they infect. Outside the living cells, viruses are dormant. Their 'life' requires invasion of a living cell.

Viruses are submicroscopic.

A viral infection is systemic. Viruses infect a host cell and then replicate. After leaving the host, they go on to infect other cells of the body.

Systemic diseases caused by viral infection include, measles, polio, AIDS, Influenza (Flu) and COVID-19.

VS

Bacteria

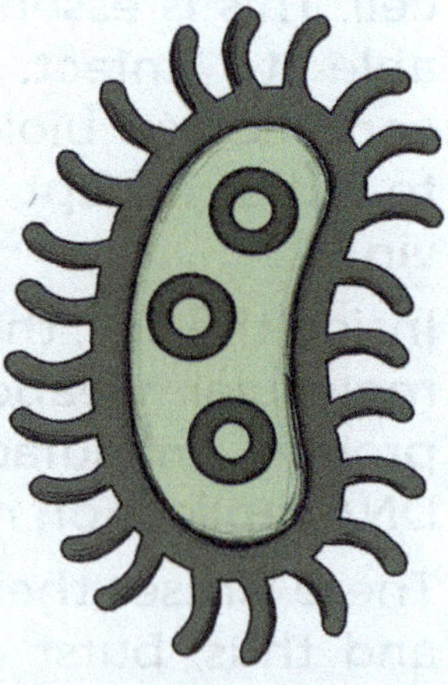

Bacteria are living organisms

Bacterium are single cell organisms that can generate energy, make their own food, move and reproduce. This is why bacteria can live in many places such as soil, plants, water, and the human body.

Bacteria are huge compared to viruses.

A bacterial infection is usually localized to a particular part of the body. The infection can be either a result of the bacteria or by the by-products of the bacteria, such as endotoxins.

Bacterial diseases include pneumonia, tuberculosis, tetanus and even food poisoning.

2 Journey into the Body

- The Highway of Oxygen
- The Main Stage

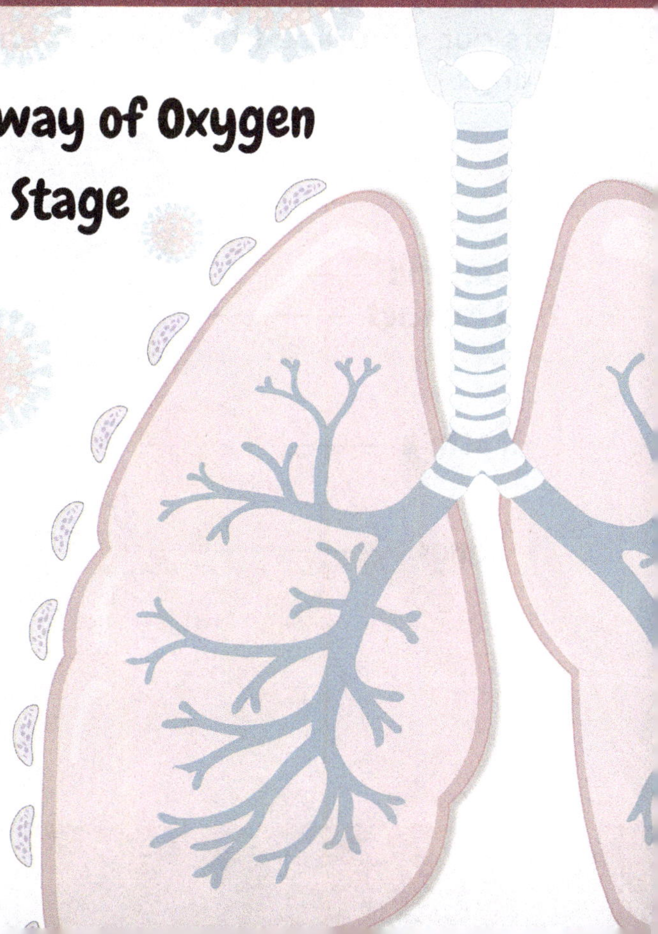

Journey into the Body

A virus infects our body by entering healthy cells. In the case of SARS-CoV-2, it starts its journey from the eyes, nose, or mouth. Evidence suggests that its destinations are the intestines, kidneys, liver, spleen, heart, and where it has the most catastrophic effect, the lungs. In the earlier days of infection, this coronavirus invades the cells which are located in the lining of the airways. These cells are the first line of defense for any outside debris, pollen, or foreign molecules.

The Highway of Oxygen

The respiratory tract is our body's highway of oxygen. Air begins in the external environment, and moves into our nasal or oral cavities. It shuttles its way down our respiratory tract, which is the upside-down tree inside our body. The air then enters our windpipe (the trachea), and continues down into our lungs.

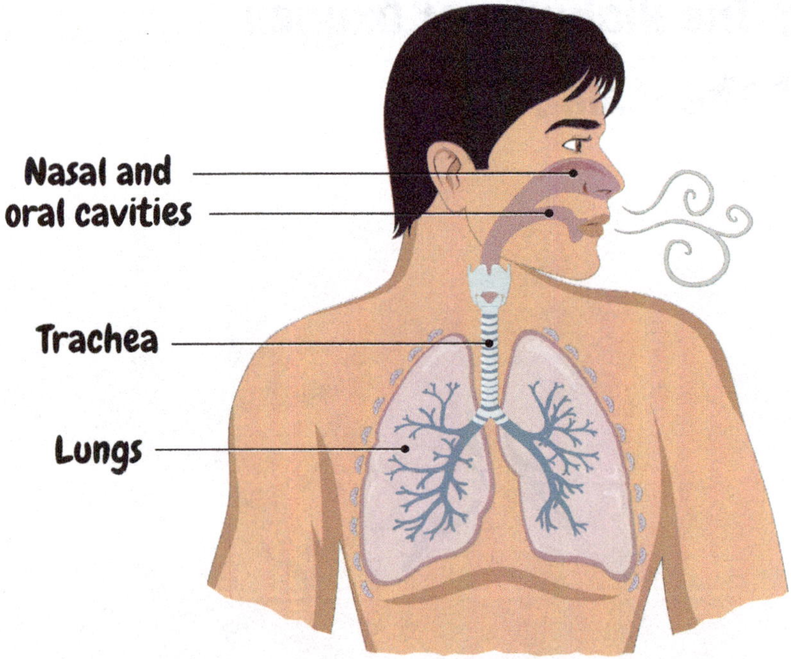

As air travels down, the trachea bifurcates at the 'carina'. Here, the air decides to go either right or left into the primary, to the secondary, and to the tertiary extensions of our windpipe, the bronchi. These bronchi split once again into even smaller paths called bronchioles, which consist of the area we are most interested in, that is, 'the alveoli'. This is the main stage!

The Lungs

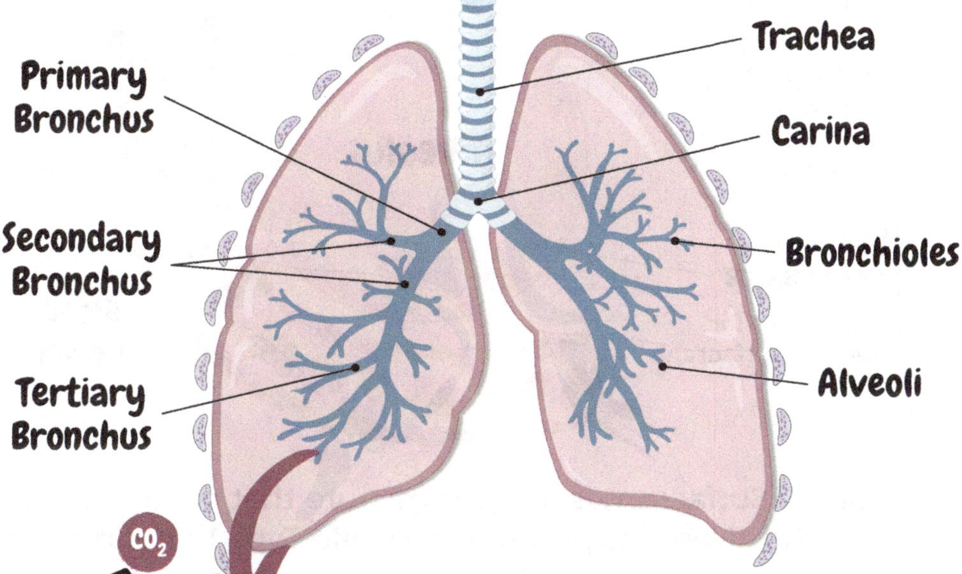

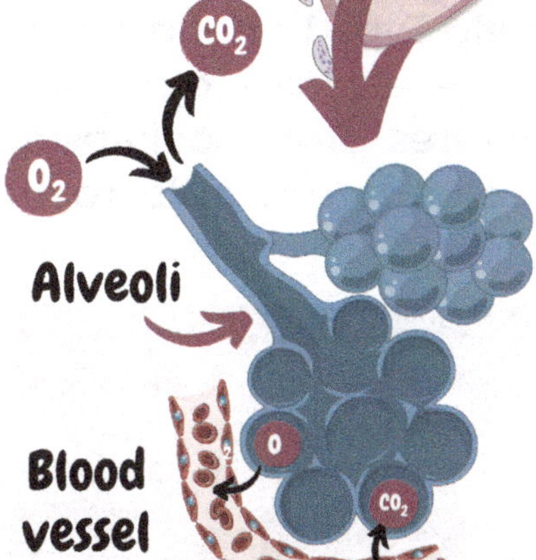

When healthy lungs inhale, they fill with oxygen, together with their 480 million tiny air sacs called the alveoli. These air sacs get rid of carbon dioxide when we exhale, and pass oxygen into the blood vessels.

The Main Stage

SARS-CoV-2 invades mainly the alveolar cells found in our alveoli, thus giving rise to the respiratory complications that we will discuss.

One alveolus is made up of two types of alveolar cells: Type 1 pneumocytes and Type 2 pneumocytes.

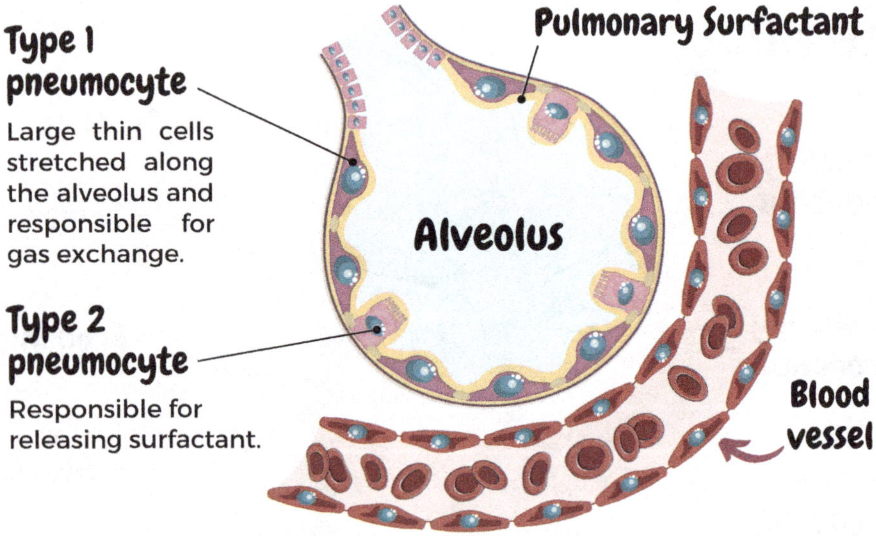

Pulmonary Surfactant is a liquid mixture that coats the inner lining of the alveoli. Its purpose is to help Type 1 pneumocytes carry out their function of keeping the alveolus open and preventing these balloon-like structures from collapsing when we breathe. A collapsed alveolus is not able to be blown up again.

Bacterial pneumonia in preterm and term newborn babies can cause problems with the functioning of pulmonary surfactant. Any disruption in surfactant function makes breathing very difficult for these infants.

3 The Invasion Begins

- **SARS-CoV-2 loves our Alveoli**
  - **Invasion and Replication**
- **What do we do when we're hurt? We call for aid.**

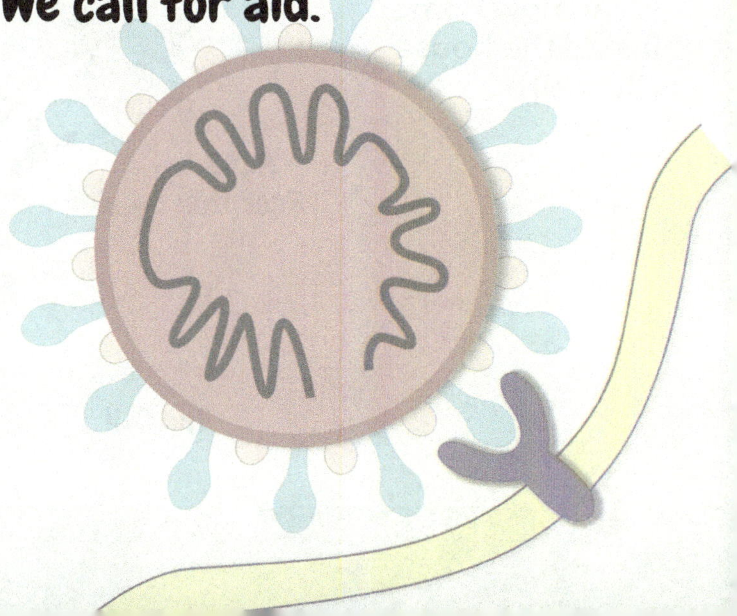

The Invasion Begins

Even just a few coronaviruses can cause a dramatic situation inside the body. SARS-CoV-2 is very similar to previous human respiratory coronaviruses, and has all the same genetic equipment which can cause a major outbreak, starting in our bodies, and moving on to the rest of the world. The lungs are lined with billions of alveolar cells, which the SARS-CoV-2 particle connects to via a specific receptor on its victim's cell. From here, it injects its genetic material for it to replicate.

SARS-CoV-2 loves our Alveoli

Like other coronaviruses, SARS-CoV-2 particles are spherical, and the key to infection are the spikes! The Spike proteins (S) of SARS-CoV-2 latch onto the cell's receptor called the angiotensin-converting enzyme 2 (ACE2), which are on surfaces of type 2 pneumocytes in the alveoli. This process is carried out the same way as the SARS outbreak in 2002.

So once the 'key' (the S protein) of SARS-CoV-2 clings to the door lock (ACE2), guess what?

It can now come inside the house (the cell).

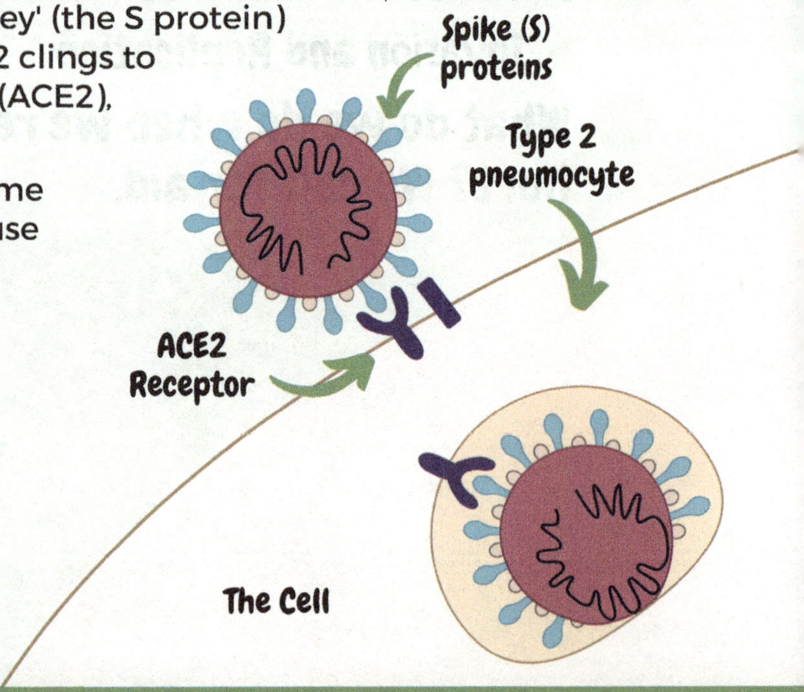

When attached, the SARS-CoV-2 particle undergoes a structural change that allows its viral membrane to fuse with the target cell's membrane. This cell is naive and unknowing; it follows the instructions from the virus, and does what the virus asks it to do, that is, copy and reassemble.

The virus binds and targets ACE2, which is a receptor and an enzyme on the surface of type 2 pneumocyte cells. Other than the lungs, the ACE2 receptors are also found on kidney, heart, and gut cells.

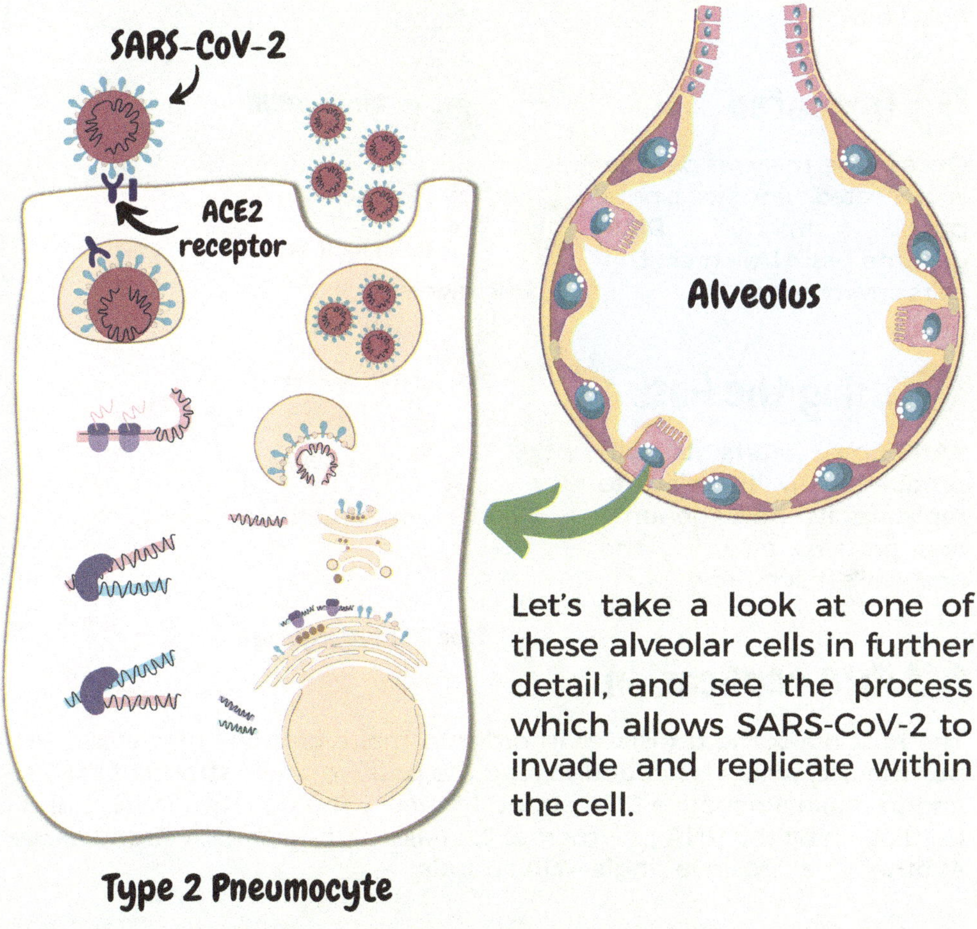

Let's take a look at one of these alveolar cells in further detail, and see the process which allows SARS-CoV-2 to invade and replicate within the cell.

The Invasion Begins

INVASION AND REPLICATION OF SARS-COV-2 INSIDE ALVEOLAR CELLS

1 Entry

It uses its spike proteins (its key) to target and bind onto the ACE2 receptor (door lock). This is the process called endocytosis. It can also enter by direct fusion of the virus envelope with the host cell.

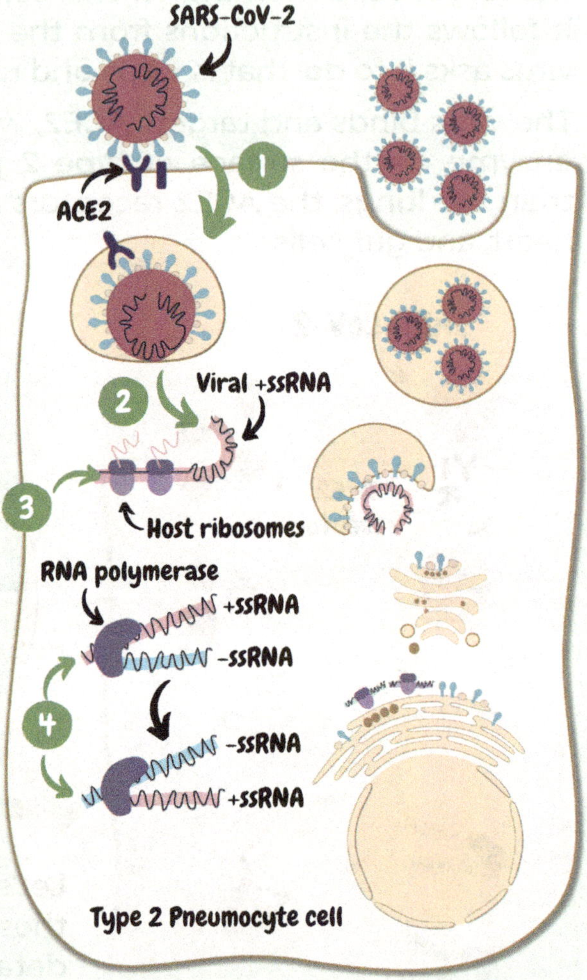

2 Uncoated

Once inside, the virus particle is uncoated, and its single positive stranded RNA genome (+ssRNA) enters the cell's environment.

3 Using the host

SARS-CoV-2 starts its self-production by its ability to replicate its new genome and proteins by using the host cell's machinery.

4 RNA replication

The host ribosome translates in order to make proteins that make RNA polymerase, which is needed to read the positive single strand of the RNA and to make a negative RNA strand (-ssRNA). The negative RNA strand is used again by the RNA polymerase to make a positive RNA strand as well as other small positive single RNA strands.

INVASION AND REPLICATION OF SARS-COV-2 INSIDE ALVEOLAR CELLS

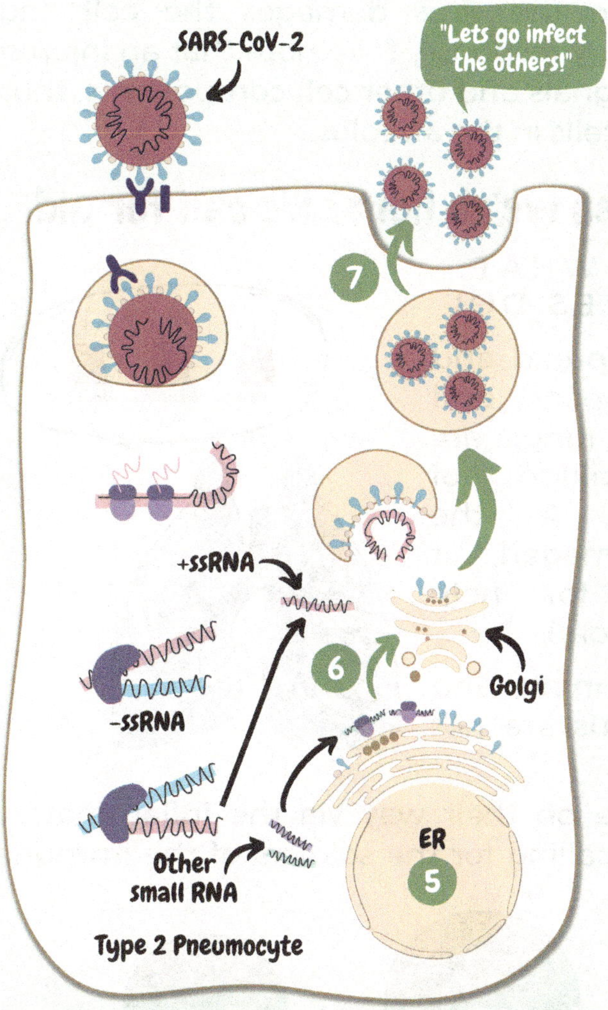

5 Structuring

The small positive RNA strands are read by the host ribosomes in the endoplasmic reticulum (ER) to help make the structural components of the virus.

6 Packaging

The ER transfers its results and other accessory proteins to the golgi apparatus. This is where everything is packaged with the positive single RNA strand in order to ship out.

7 Exit

These newly made viruses are now released via exocytosis (the process by which products of the cell are expelled out into the cell's surrounding).

Scientists and experts believe that treatments targeting ACE2 (angiotensin converting enzyme-2), could be the key to unlocking either a treatment for COVID-19 or a coronavirus vaccine.

The Invasion Begins

The cell fills up with more and more copies of the virus, until it reaches a maximum point and undergoes self-destruction. This happens because the virus damages the cell and initiates an inflammatory response. Take note that an injured alveolar cell releases signals and other cell components, thus affecting neighboring cells in the alveolus.

What do we do when we're hurt? We call for aid.

THIS IS EXACTLY WHAT OUR PNEUMOCYTES DO!

The virus begins to spread and multiply at a rapid pace, and after 7-10 days, the lungs are overwhelmed by billions of viruses infecting it. As the pneumocyte is damaged, it sends out a cry for help (inflammatory mediators).

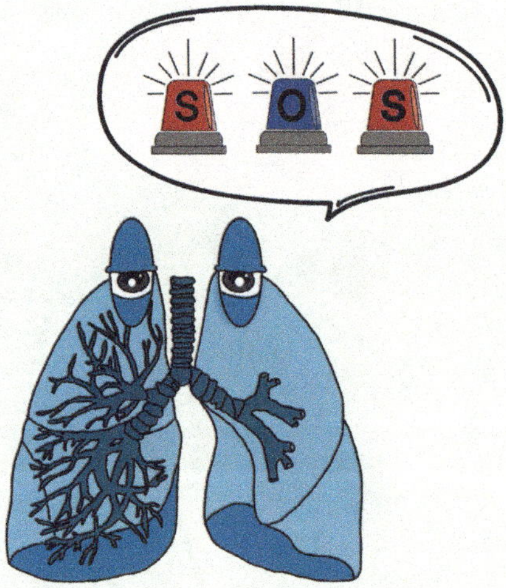

This is just the beginning, and the effects of the virus are not noticed yet.

The real problems are on their way via the inflammatory mediators, which are calling for the soldiers of the immune system.

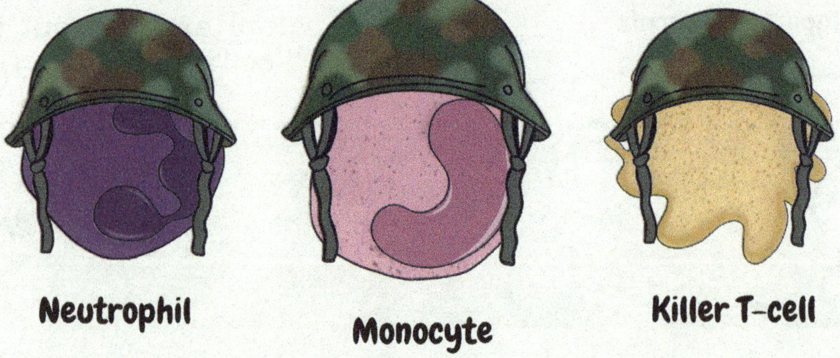

4 How the Body fights back

- The War begins
- The Troops
- The Aftermath

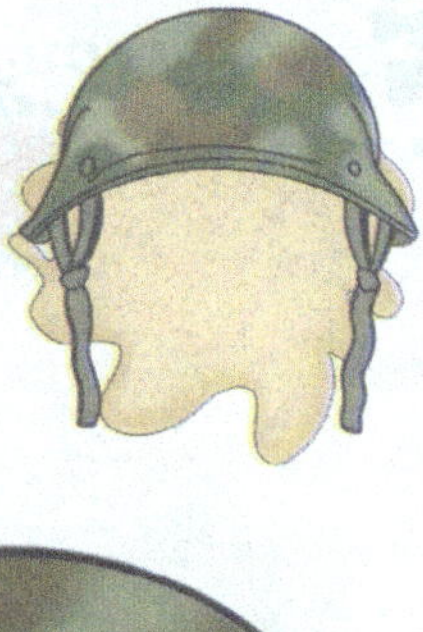

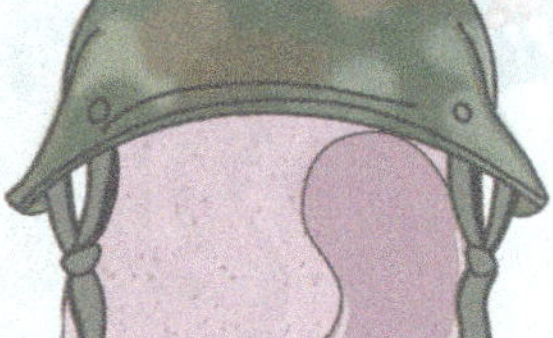

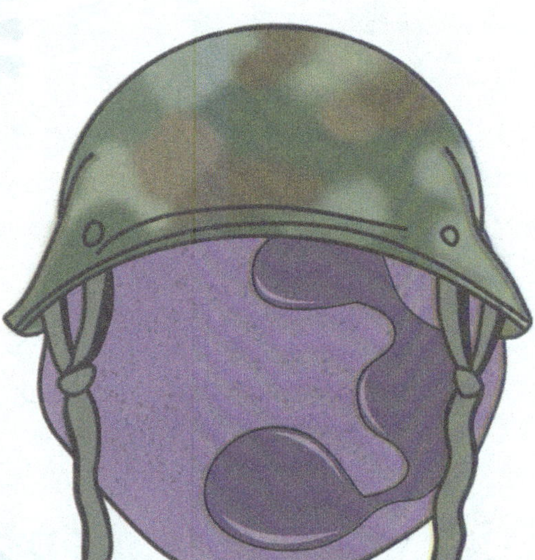

How the Body fights back

The immune system is there to protect us, but it can actually be pretty dangerous to our body, and needs tight regulation. As immune cells pour into the lungs to fight the virus, SARS-CoV-2 infects some of them and creates havoc in the body. The cells obviously can't see or speak, but they communicate mostly through tiny information proteins called cytokines.

The War begins

When injured alveolar cells burst, they release proteins, intracellular components, and SARS-CoV-2 particles that were inside of them. The cell also issues an inflammatory response by releasing interferons (signals to nearby unaffected cells to increase the anti-viral defense) and cytokines. The messages by cytokines trigger and stimulate our nerve endings which are responsible for initiating the cough reflex. This is the reason why people with COVID-19 have a **'dry cough'**.

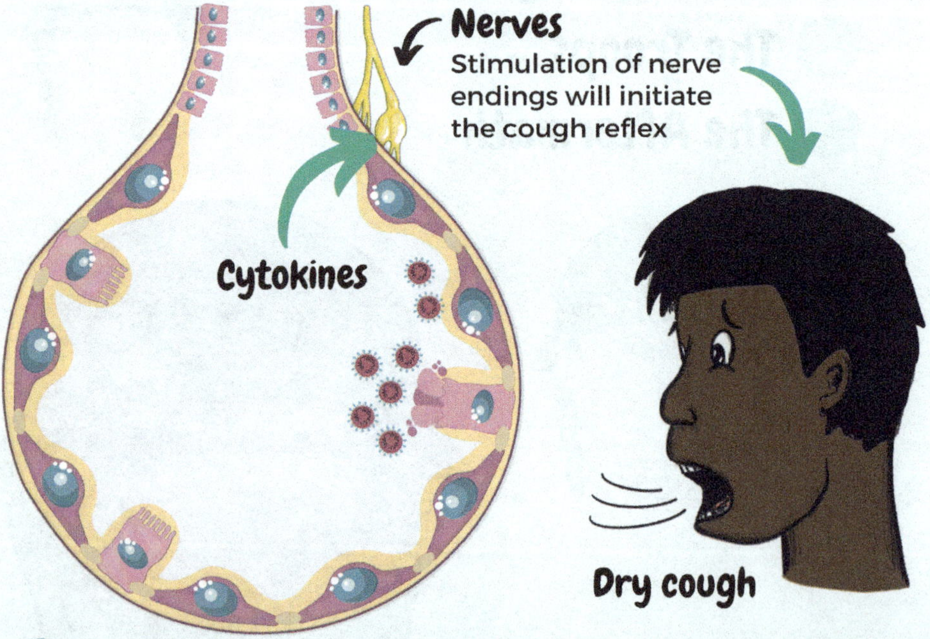

The Troops

The cells in the alveoli send signals (inflammatory mediators) to the bloodstream, and start recruiting the soldiers for the battle, our body's immune cells. These immune soldiers come to the site of damage stimulating an inflammatory response to try and heal the site. The soldiers include neutrophils, killer T-cells, and monocytes.

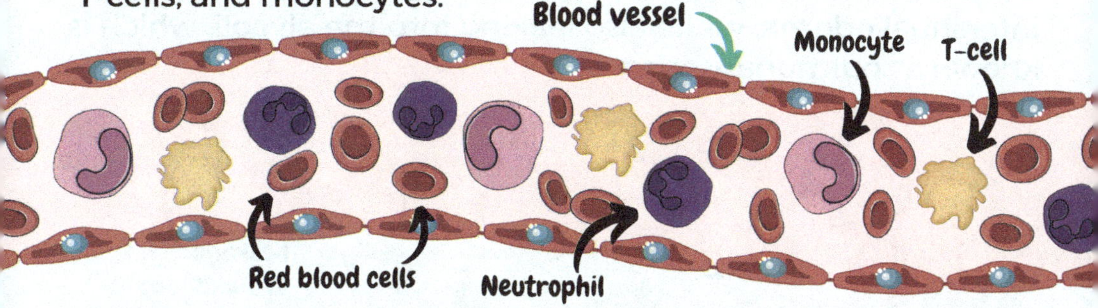

The neutrophils, which are the go-to cell to kill invaders, come over to the site in huge numbers. They are known to pump out enzymes that destroy the invaders. Killer T-cells however, work differently. There job usually is to order infected cells to commit controlled suicide. The over reacted response from the immune cells consequently cause damage to healthy cells as well. Below is a typical 3 step process of a killer T-cell response:

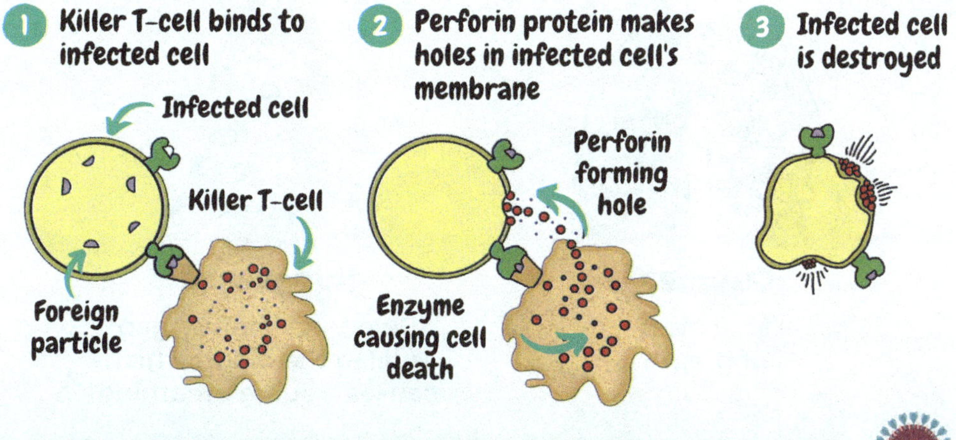

The Aftermath

As a result of the inflammation, our small blood vessels called capillaries, which surround our alveoli, become dilated. Cells which make up the capillaries stretch and form spaces between one another. Consequently, the capillaries become more porous, and cause fluids to leak out and fill the space between the lung tissue and the capillaries, known as interstitial edema, while also leaking into the alveoli, which is known as pulmonary edema.

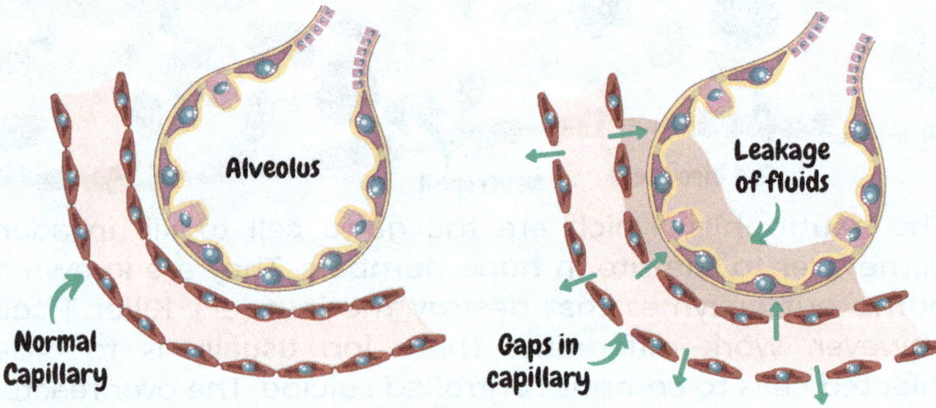

The fluid surrounding the lung tissue causes it to compress. Now the air cannot fill the lungs properly, and so, the person experiences:

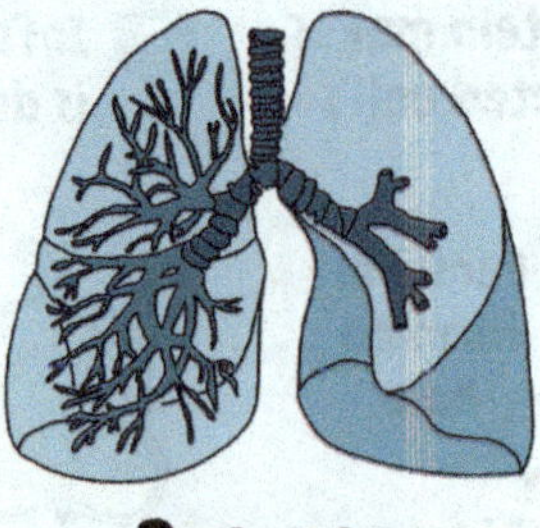

Dyspnea
Shortness of breath

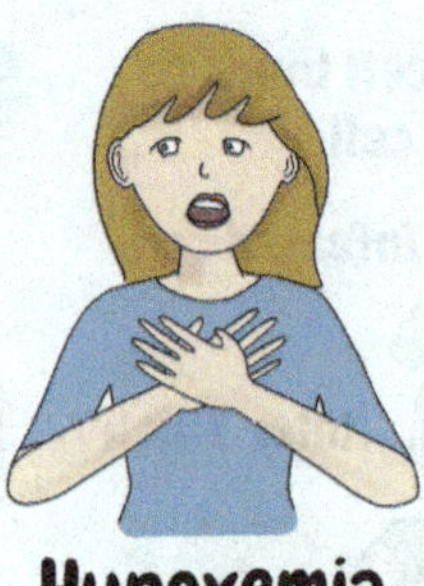

Hypoxemia
Below-normal oxygen level in the blood which causes trouble breathing

How the Body fights back

While neutrophils are great for what they do, which is to engulf bacteria and other debris around the area, they can actually be detrimental because they release chemicals which damage the pneumocytes and other neighboring alveolar cells, thus producing less surfactant. Less production of surfactant means that the alveoli can easily collapse and leave us gasping for air.

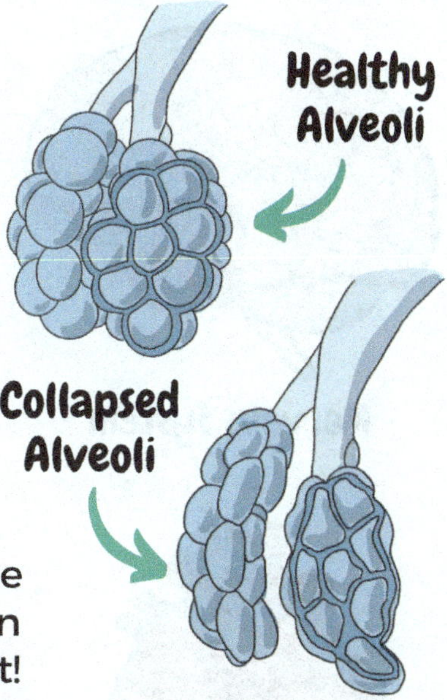

Now, while all this is happening in the lungs, there is also a multi-organ response. Our brain is stimulated to act!

The brain now has to tell the lungs to breathe more in order to increase oxygen levels in the blood.

And it tells the heart to pump faster to deliver oxygen to the body.

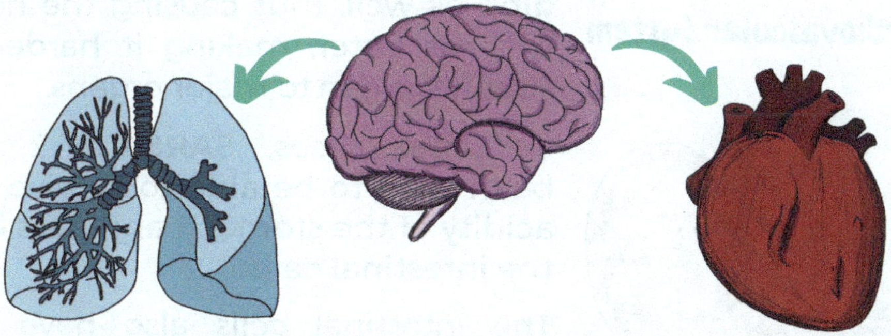

This is why people who have **hypoxemia** can also have abnormally rapid breathing, also known as **tachypnea**. Furthermore, people experience a rapid heartbeat (more than 100 times per minute), which is referred to as **tachycardia**.

How the Body fights back

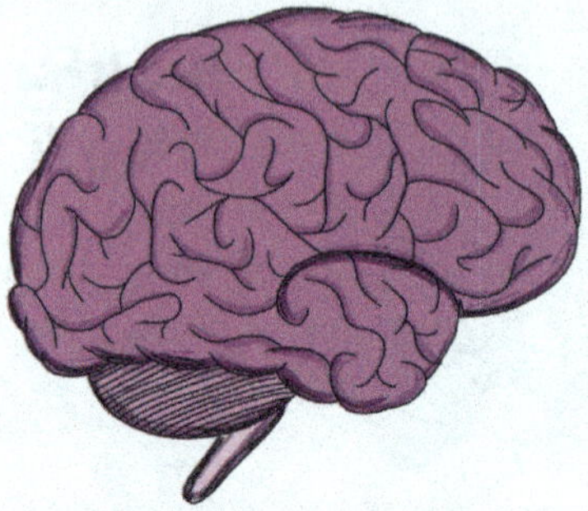

Nervous System

All the chemicals released during the war find their way into our blood transport system, where they can reach the brain.

Inside the brain, we have our body's thermostat, the hypothalamus. The chemicals cause the hypothalamus to increase our body temperature, and therefore, we experience **fever** and **headache.**

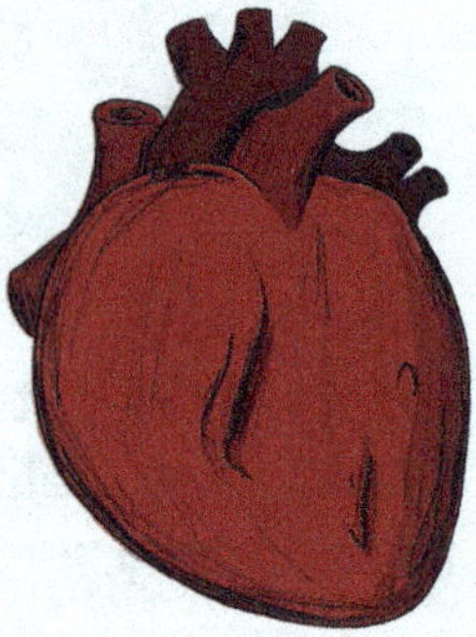

Cardiovascular System

The virus causes direct damage to the lungs, and its inflammatory response puts stress on the heart in two ways:

Firstly, by infecting the lungs, the blood oxygen levels drop, and secondly, the inflammatory effects of the virus cause the blood pressure to drop as well, thus causing the heart to beat faster, making it harder to supply oxygen to major organs.

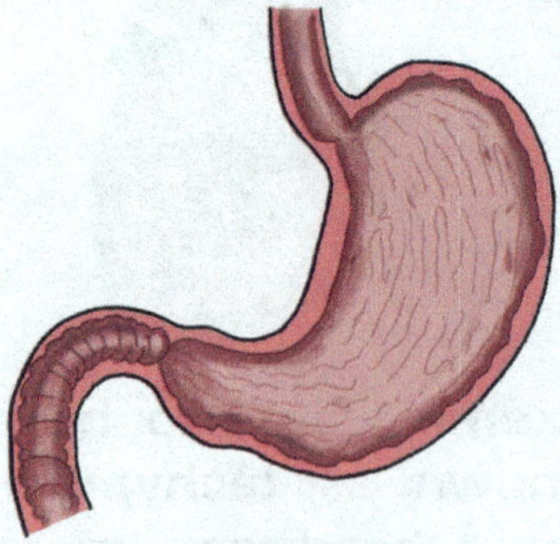

GI System

In some cases, SARS-CoV-2 has been seen to be able to survive the acidity of the stomach and pass into the intestinal cells.

The intestinal cells also have the ACE2 receptor for the entry of the virus. Therefore, the virus can multiply and infect the gastro-intestinal system, causing symptoms of **diarrhea, nausea,** and **vomiting.**

How the Body fights back

Overall, as more and more immune cells arrive to help fight off the virus, they can also create a hostile environment. These cells can cause damage to our healthy cells and, in turn, we see more healthy lung tissue die.

But not to worry, because in most cases the immune system slowly regains control. It kills the infected cells, intercepts the viruses trying to wiggle their way into new cells, and levels the playing field. Good news – recovery mode has started.

Data shows that majority of people (about 80%) infected by COVID-19 will get through it with relatively mild infection and some will not develop any symptoms at all. Others are seen to develop mild symptoms such as a dry cough, fever and shortness of breath. Symptoms can also include fatigue, loss of smell and taste. Around 15% individuals infected will have a severe disease and 5% are considered to have illness which is life threatening, such as: respiratory failure, shock, and multi-organ dysfunction.

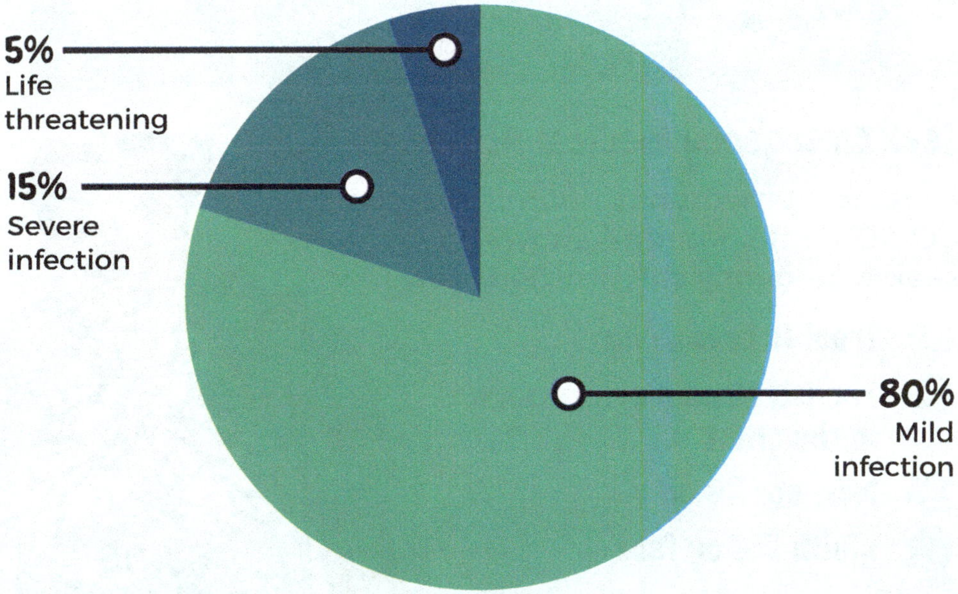

Watch for COVID-19 symptoms

Individuals can vary from a wide range of symptoms. Ranging from mild to severe illness. Symptoms may appear 2-14 days after exposure to the virus. People with these symptoms may have COVID-19:

Cough	Fever or chills	Muscle or body aches	Fatigue or lack of energy
Shortness of breath	Difficulty breathing	Headache	Loss of taste or smell
Sore throat	Congestion or runny nose	Nausea or vomiting	Diarrhea

Seek Emergency Medical Attention

Look for emergency warning signs for COVID-19. If someone shows these signs, seek emergency care immediately.

- **Trouble breathing**
- **Persistent pain or pressure in the chest**
- **New confusion**
- **Bluish lips or face**

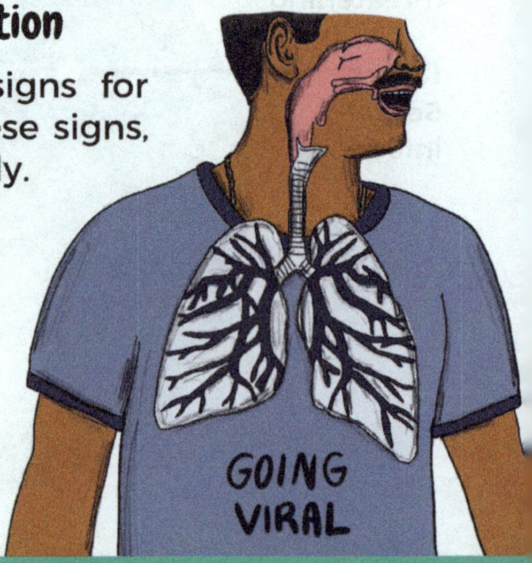

5 What happens in severe cases?

- Lungs are overwhelmed
  - What does a ventilator do?
- COVID-19 effects on the lungs and body
  - Pneumonia
  - ARDS
  - Sepsis
- Who is at risk or most vulnerable?

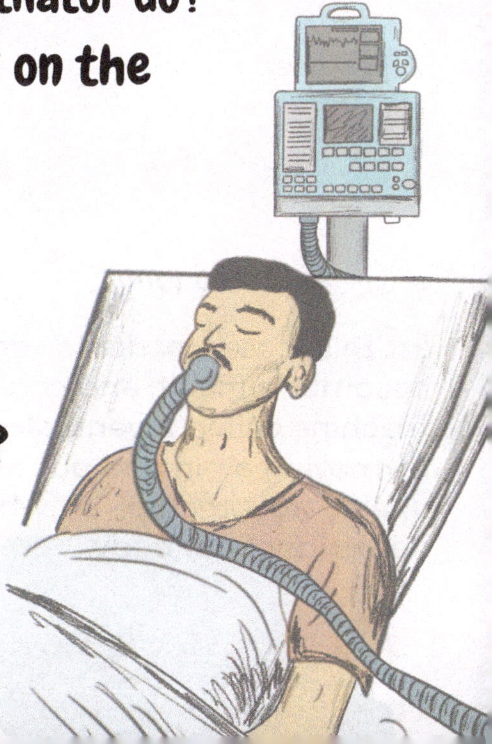

What happens in severe cases?

The elderly and those with underlying health conditions, such as cardiovascular and chronic respiratory diseases, are at increased risk for more critical cases of COVID-19. Most people infected by SARS-CoV-2 see its effects in the upper respiratory tract, such as the throat and nose; however, in the chance of severe cases, the virus travels down the respiratory tract and finds a spot in the lungs.

Lungs are overwhelmed

If we look at the critical level, millions of epithelial cells have died, and with them, the protective lining of the lungs is compromised. This means that the alveoli, our small air sacs which transport oxygen to our body, can be further infected by foreign pathogens other than SARS-CoV-2.

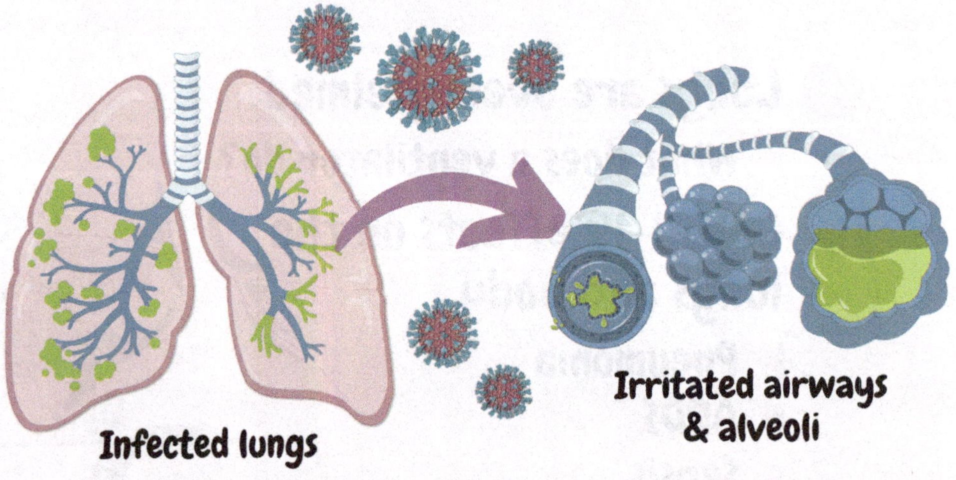

In this case, patients develop lung disease, respiration becomes difficult, and could even fail. Patients now require a machine called a ventilator, which provides aided breathing by moving air in and out of the lungs. It is used when we are unable to breathe, or when breathing can not meet the demands of our body.

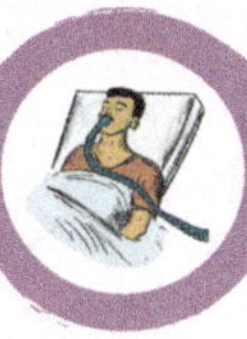

What does a ventilator do?

Less than 10% of individuals with COVID-19 become critically ill. However, 1 in 4 may need a ventilator to breathe.

What is a ventilator?

A machine which mechanically pumps oxygen into the airways and takes the breaths for us.

How long do we need it?

It helps us survive until our lungs are once again capable of breathing on their own. It is not used as a cure for COVID-19.

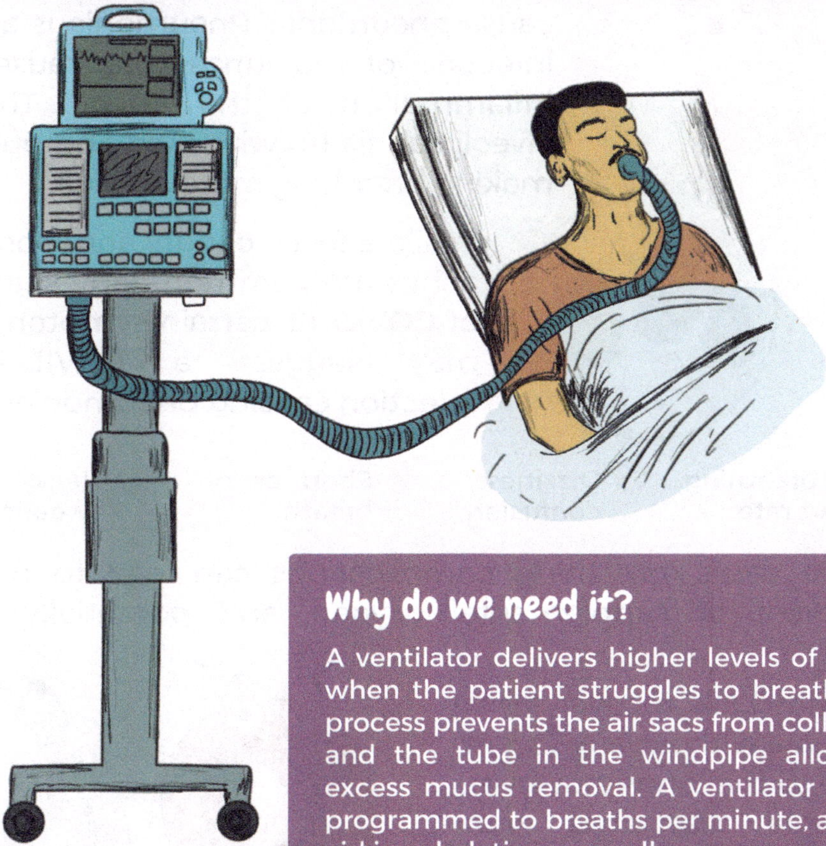

Why do we need it?

A ventilator delivers higher levels of oxygen when the patient struggles to breathe. The process prevents the air sacs from collapsing, and the tube in the windpipe allows for excess mucus removal. A ventilator can be programmed to breaths per minute, and can aid in exhalations as well.

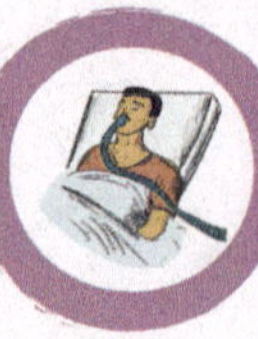

What happens in severe cases?

COVID-19 effects on the lungs and body

Serious effects of SARS-CoV-2 are seen at the lower respiratory tract level. Here, the infection has reached the lungs, and symptoms can become more severe. The lungs, which are the production factory of oxygen, can become inflamed, and matters can quickly worsen, leading to pneumonia.

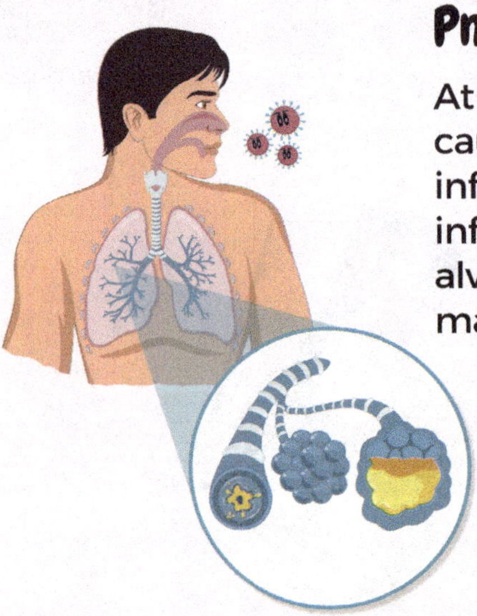

Pneumonia

At the critical level, SARS-CoV-2 can cause pneumonia. Pneumonia is an infection of the lungs that causes inflammation of the alveoli. The alveoli can fill up with fluid and pus, making breathing more difficult

While a fever, cough, and, body aches are common early signs of COVID-19, certain symptoms may suggest a COVID-19 infection causing pneumonia:

- Rapid breathing or heart rate
- Dizziness/ confusion
- Shortness of breath
- Heavy sweating

In severe cases, breathing complications can lead to the requirement of supplemental oxygen, and potentially a ventilator.

Most individuals recover from pneumonia without any severe damage to the lungs; however, pneumonia associated with COVID-19 may be more severe.

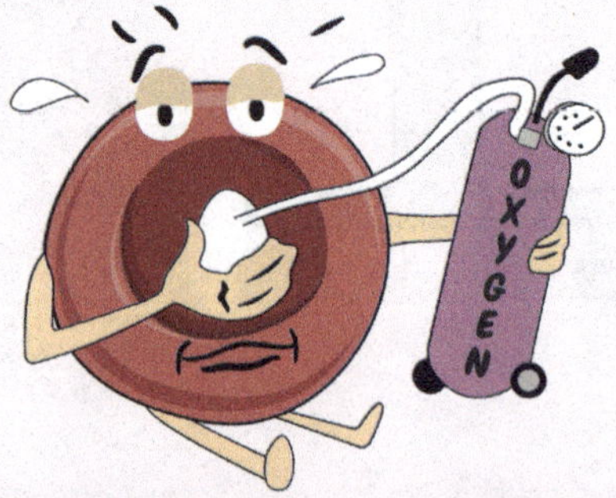

What happens in severe cases?

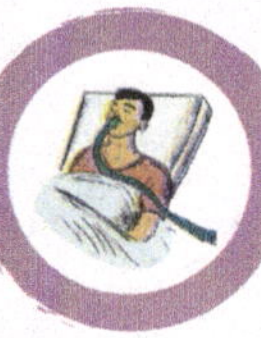

Acute Respiratory Distress Syndrome (ARDS)

When lung damage and inflammation is so severe and pneumonia progresses, fluid builds up around and within the lungs, leading to a form of lung failure called Acute Respiratory Distress Syndrome (ARDS). The individual exhibits hypoxemia, a below-normal oxygen level in the blood, and experiences shortness of breath. In some cases, patients with ARDS are unable to breathe on their own, and require ventilator support to breathe.

Normal Alveoli

Normal gas exchange, and thin alveolar walls. Easy uptake of oxygen and release of carbon dioxide.

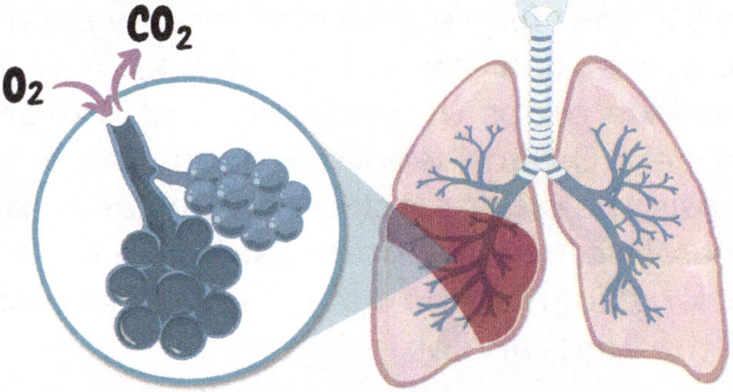

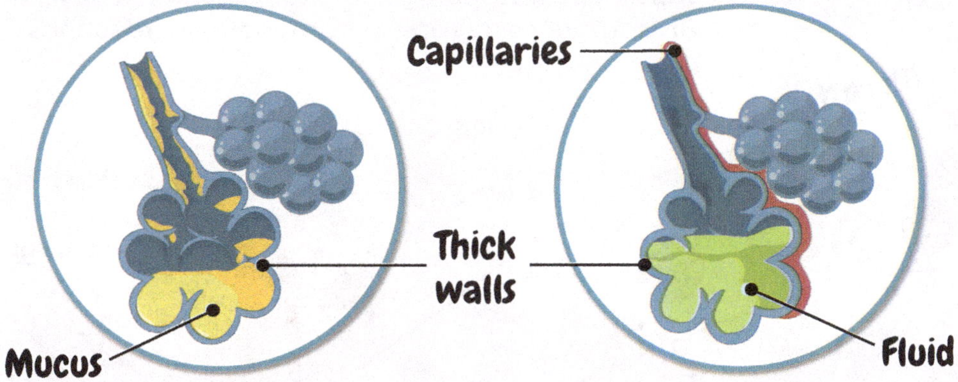

Pneumonia

Thick and irritated alveolar walls, with accumulation of mucus and inflammatory cells.

ARDS and Pneumonia

Fluid releasing from capillaries, filling the alveolar space, and preventing gas exchange.

What happens in severe cases?

When the body is infected, our immune system is fighting at its full capacity, while making millions of antiviral weapons. Since this virus is multiplying rapidly, the body is overwhelmed. The virus begins to enter the blood and starts an entire takeover. If all this occurs, death is very likely.

Sepsis

A severe consequence of COVID-19 can be sepsis. This is when the infection of SARS-CoV-2 uses the body's bloodstream to spread and reach tissue at further locations. The virus has the ability to inflict severe damage everywhere it goes and the outcome can be septic shock. This is when the blood pressure drops dramatically and the organs are starved for oxygen. Organs work together like a team; however, with sepsis, the organs lack communication between one another. Therefore, we see entire systems in the body fail one after the other. Patients who survive sepsis have severe lasting damage to the lungs and organ systems.

Sepsis causes damage to vital organs because the virus trigger's complex immunologic reactions in the body.

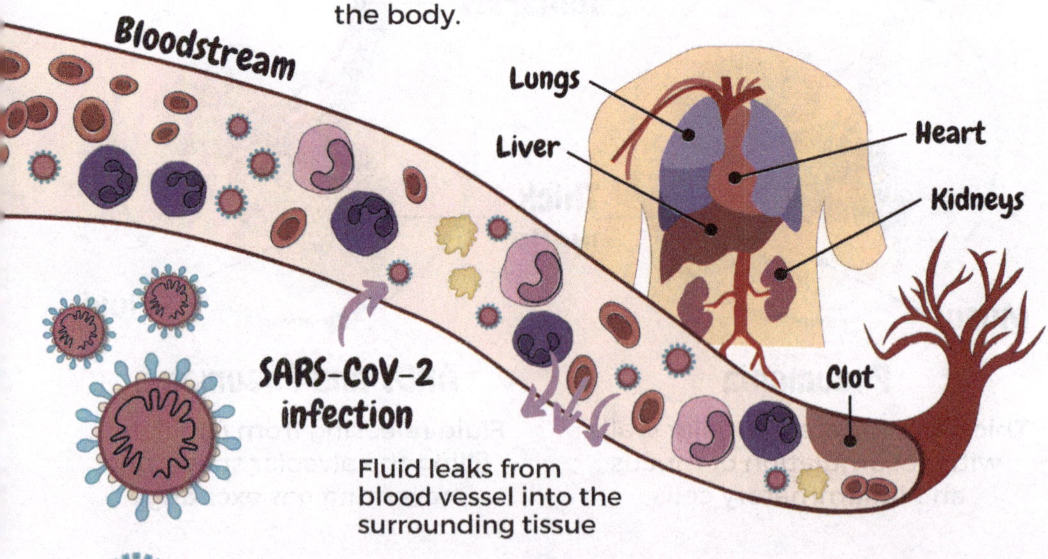

What happens in severe cases?

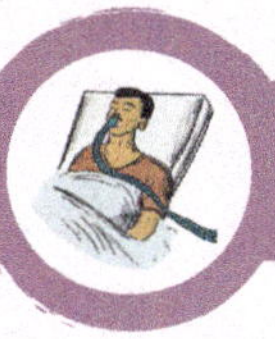

It is unlikely that young and healthy individuals die from SARS-CoV-2, but they could develop a chronic lung condition called Pulmonary Fibrosis, which occurs when the lung tissue is damaged and scarred.

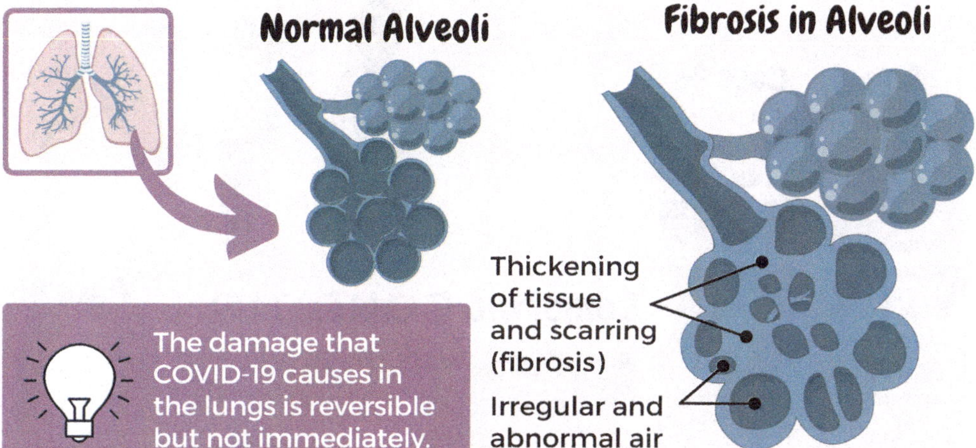

The damage that COVID-19 causes in the lungs is reversible but not immediately.

Although the lung tissue heals slowly, it can take several years for normal function to return. Continuous treatment and therapy will be required for individuals post- COVID-19. Your medical provider may even suggest pulmonary rehabilitation to ease you into your daily activities, especially if your illness was severe or critical.

Pulmonary rehab gives you hope to regain strength and enjoy a more active lifestyle. The program improves lung function, reduces symptom severity and improves quality of life.

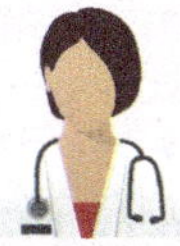

Education about symptoms, condition, medication and oxygen

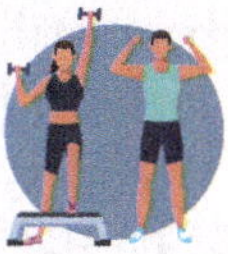

Supervised exercise classes and instruction for breathing techniques

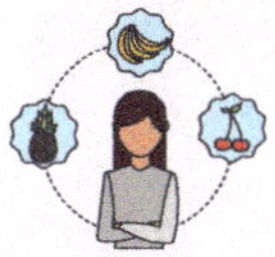

Nutritional counseling and guided emotional health support

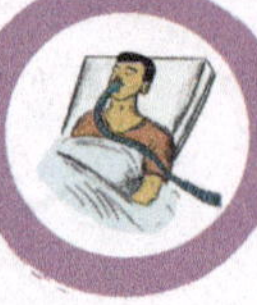

What happens in severe cases?

Who is at risk or most vulnerable?

It can be seen that the elderly and those with comorbidities are at highest risk, while individuals under 60 have a small percentage of fatality.

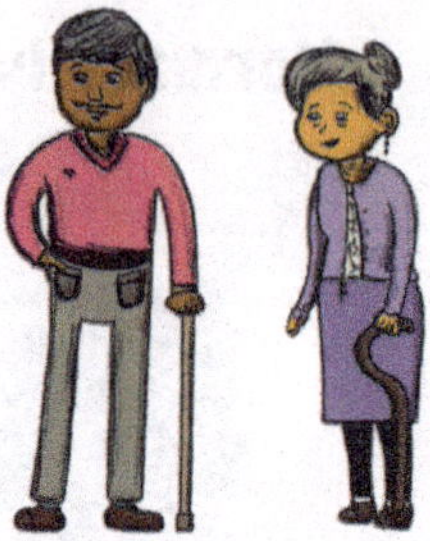

Age YEARS	Case % FATALITY RATE
>80	14.8
70-79	8.0
60-69	3.6
50-59	1.3
40-49	0.4
30-39	0.2
20-29	0.2
10-19	0.2
0-9	---

Comorbid CONDITION	Case % FATALITY RATE
Cardiovascular disease	10.5
Diabetes	7.3
Chronic Lung disease	6.3
Hypertension	6.0
Cancer (Any type)	5.6
No pre-existing conditions	0.9

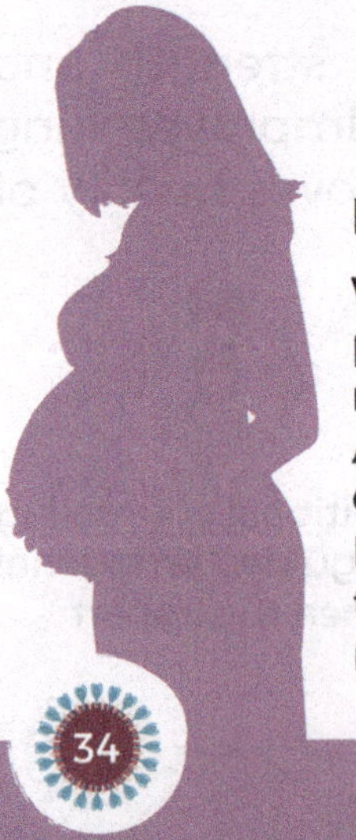

PREGNANT WOMEN

While research is still pending, it seems that healthy pregnant people are NOT at high risk. So far, there are no cases of intrauterine transmission of COVID-19. Additionally, a group of mothers who were positive for COVID-19 were tested for this virus in their breast milk. It was found, in terms of breastfeeding, that the main transmission is still through respiratory droplets, and is not detected in breast milk.

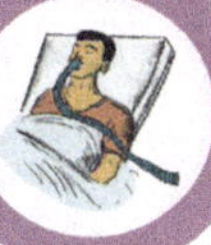

Common Cold vs. Influenza (Flu) vs. COVID-19

COVID-19, Influenza, and the Common Cold are all respiratory illnesses; yet, all three are caused by different viruses. COVID-19, as explained earlier, is caused by SARS-CoV-2. The common cold is caused by numerous viruses, mainly rhinovirus (30–80%), picornavirus, and influenza viruses (10-15%), including human coronaviruses (≈15%). Frequently, more than one virus is present.

Influenza, also known as the 'flu', is caused by influenza viruses Types A, B, C, and/or D. The COVID-19 outbreak has not been the only pandemic we have had to deal with. In 1918, the influenza pandemic was one of the most severe pandemics recorded in recent history, which was caused by an H1N1 virus (Type A Influenza Virus) with genes of avian origin. Although there is no universal consensus regarding the origins of the virus, it spread worldwide during 1918-1919. It is estimated that about one-third of the world's population became infected, while the number of deaths was estimated to be at least 50 million worldwide.

What does the COVID-19 pandemic and the Influenza pandemic have in common?

Like the COVID-19 pandemic, the Influenza pandemic did not have a vaccine at the time. Additionally, similarly to COVID-19, Influenza did not have medication to treat or prevent it. Therefore, control efforts worldwide were limited to non-pharmaceutical interventions, such as isolation, quarantine, good personal hygiene, use of disinfectants, and limitations of public gatherings. On the other hand, the common cold is milder than the flu and COVID-19, and thankfully, colds do not result in serious health problems, such as, pneumonia, bacterial infections, or hospitalizations. Both the flu and COVID-19 can however have very serious complications.

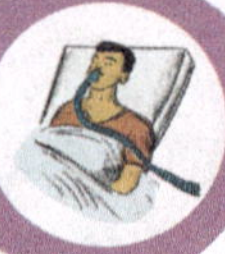

What happens in severe cases?

Symptoms	Common Cold	Influenza (Flu)	COVID-19 (Coronavirus)
Fever	Rare	Common	Common
Headache	Rare	Common	Sometimes
Body aches	Mild	Common	Sometimes
Sneezing	Common	Sometimes	Been reported
Sore throat	Common	Sometimes	Sometimes
Diarrhea	Rare	Sometimes	Rare
Cough	Mild	Common	Common (dry)
Shortness of breath	No	Rare	Mild/moderate infection
Difficulty breathing	No	In severe infection	In severe infection
Runny or stuffy nose	Common	Sometimes	Rare
Fatigue, weakness	Mild	Common	Sometimes
Symptom onset	Gradual	Abrupt	Gradual
Incubation period	1-3 days	1-4 days	1-14 days

6 Understanding COVID-19 vaccines

- **Development of a vaccine**
  - **Safety and Efficacy**
  - **Phases**
- **How do the vaccines work?**
  - **Moderna NIAID, Pfizer BioNTech**
  - **Oxford/AstraZeneca**
- **Booster Shots and Additional Doses**
- **Self-Care**

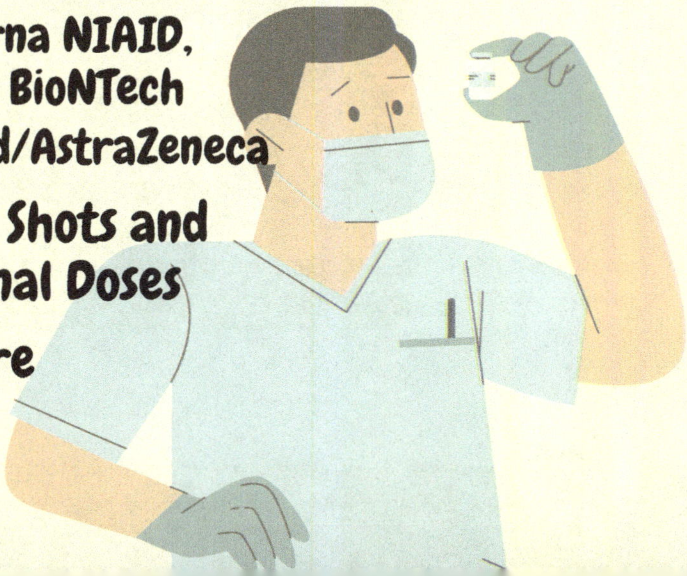

Understanding COVID-19 vaccines

Important

Those affected by the virus should seek and receive care to relieve the symptoms. If you, or a loved one, have a serious illness, then it's best to seek medical attention immediately and be hospitalized. Most affected individuals see their symptoms subside.

COVID-19 vaccines

We will discuss primarily the three vaccines that are being funded by Operation Warp Speed in the United States. It includes the Moderna NIAID, Pfizer BioNTech, and the Oxford/AstraZeneca vaccine. We'll begin by understanding how these vaccines are developed, the particular phases and stages they must go through. Then we'll explain the mechanism of action of how these vaccines actually work in our body.

How about using antibiotics to prevent or treat COVID-19?

Antibiotics do NOT work against viruses, they only work on bacterial infections. COVID-19 is caused by a virus. You should NOT use antibiotics as any form of prevention or treatment of COVID-19.

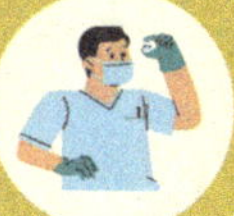

Development of a vaccine

SAFETY AND EFFICACY

Vaccine development requires stages and phases that vaccines must go through to receive FDA approval or emergency use authorization. There are two primary goals when vaccines are developed during these stages. The first goal is safety, which is the highest priority during development. It is critical to make sure that any side effects observed on patients, that received the vaccine during trials, aren't developing any serious or deadly side effects related to the vaccine.

The second goal is efficacy. Efficacy can be interpreted as the efficacy of the vaccine to prevent disease or the efficacy of the vaccine to prevent infection. Therefore we ask the two questions: Is this vaccine protective against disease? Or, is it protective against infection? It is important to establish this distinction because the disease, COVID-19 which is caused by SARS-CoV-2, can present with symptoms ranging from mild, moderate, to severe (hospitalized on ventilator or ECMO machine), or the patient could be completely asymptomatic.

Therefore when measuring efficacy we measure to see if the vaccine is effective against preventing the severity of the disease, or can it prevent asymptomatic infections and those individuals who are spreading the disease. There is still more to understand regarding this, however the primary focus for researchers is on the severity of the disease.

When we start a vaccine, what are the phases that it has to go through? And what is being tested to meet the goals of safety and efficacy?

Phases

It starts with the pre-clinical phase in which scientists will do animal testing. After, if animal testing is safe and effective, testing will move onto human trials. Human trials are placed into three phases. Phase 1 is a small population size asking the question, Is it safe and effective? If yes, we move onto phase 2 which is a larger population size. Still safe and effective? We move onto a larger population size for Phase 3. Now if all the population sizes are safe and effective, it can be sent over for FDA approval. In the case of COVID-19 pandemic the studies were sent for Emergency Use Authorization. Following these phases and trials there are peer reviewed studies that are conducted to follow up on the study.

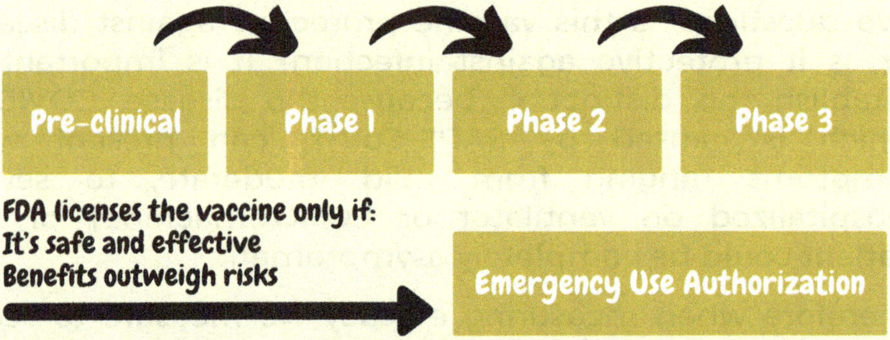

PRE-CLINICAL (ANIMAL TESTING)

During this phase the vaccine is being given to animals (mice for example). We will look for side effects, such as anything from skin irritation, fever, fatigue, or death. Also, efficacy is being monitored. After administering the vaccine to the mice, we will see if the mice are developing any antibodies, and if so, are there a certain amount of antibodies?

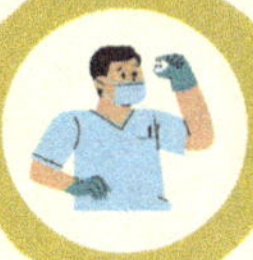

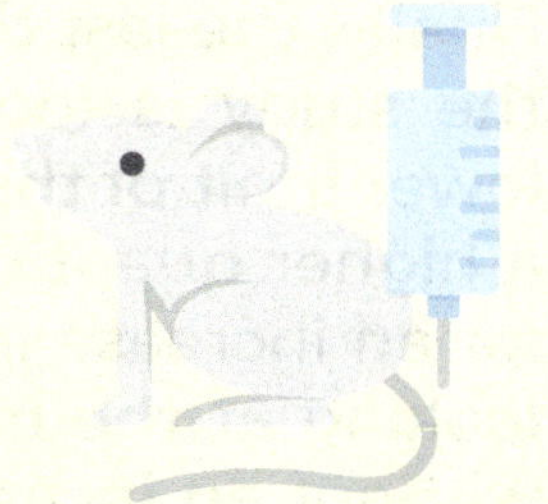

Next we'll look if these antibodies are effective in combating the SARS-CoV-2 virus.

The mice are infected with the virus and monitored to see if the vaccine that is administered is preventing the disease.

After giving the vaccine to the animals, looking at the side effects, monitoring the efficacy by antibody production, noticing the binding or the lack thereof to the pathogen, and finally seeing if there is a prevention of disease - if after all these studies have been conducted only then could you move onto phase 1-3.

PHASE 1 (HEALTHY INDIVIDUALS)

In phase 1 the vaccine is being administered to humans and being tested. But, it is given to a small sample size, which is generally less than 100 participants. During this phase it is important to have healthy humans without any comorbidities or underlying illness. This is because If they do get sick, it is from an illness rather than the vaccine that you're testing on them. Next is to see if the vaccine is causing any side effects (skin irritation, fever, fatigue, death, etc).

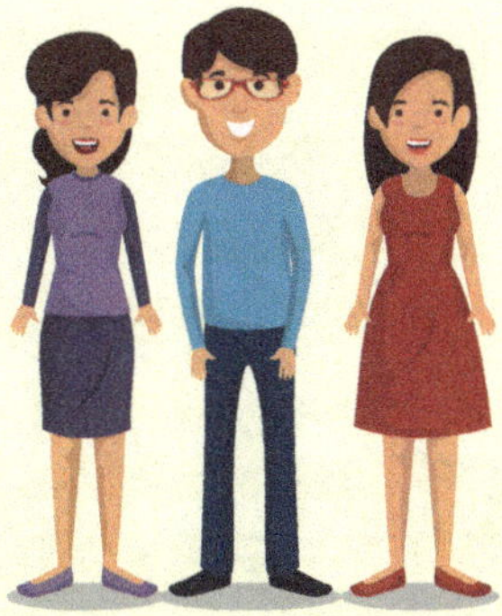

Usually less than 100 people, and monitoring for safety at multiple doses.

Finally, the last thing that is being tested is dosage. For this, the study is looking to understand the upper limit and lower limit of the dose. Upper limit is the administration of a higher quantity of the dose to review the potential risks for an increase in side effects. The upper limit is essentially looking at the highest dosage that could be administered without an inclination of side effects. In comparison, lower limits are looked at to see if a lower dosage is enough to trigger the antibody response, or if there is a decreased antibody response - in this case the vaccine won't be effective. The study tries to get in between these limits for the optimal dosage. If phase 1 runs smoothly, the study moves onto phase 2.

PHASE 2 (MATCHING DEMOGRAPHICS)

Vaccine is still being administered to humans but the number of participants increases to a moderate sample size, about 100 - 1000 participants. Unlike phase 1 where the participants were healthy individuals, in phase 2 the goal is to begin matching to the demographics of the population that the vaccine will be administered to. For example, matching to age (generally 18 and above), race, gender, and underlying comorbidities (lung disease, heart disease, cancer, etc).

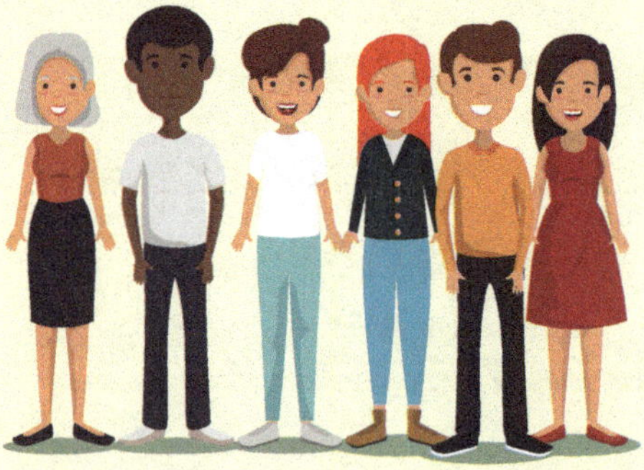

Therefore during phase 2, the sample size will include various demographics. For example those that are older, younger, asian, african american, healthy, with disease, without disease, etc.

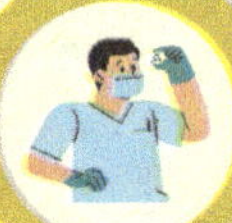

During phase 2 the side effects are still being monitored and we are looking to see if the dosage we determined in phase 1 is effective.

PHASE 3 (LARGE SAMPLE SIZE)

Vaccine continues to be tested on humans but with a large sample size, which can be anywhere from 1,000 - 100,000 participants.

During phase 3 the participants must continue to match the demographics of the population that the vaccine will be administered too. Also, the study will monitor the effectiveness of the vaccine in a real life situation. Vaccine is given to participants who are performing their regular day-to-day activities in their given environment. These participants are then closely monitored for symptoms. Some of the participants will undergo a PCR test to confirm the diagnosis and some will not be monitored for symptoms and instead be regularly swabbed to see if there is a positive reading.

In summary, we are monitoring how many participants with the vaccine who carried on with their normal daily activities, have contracted the virus. Alongside this data there is the control group who are also monitored in the real world for contracting the disease, but are given a placebo.

Once all the phases are completed and the efficacy has been studied, now it can be moved to emergency use authorization and FDA approval. This is a general understanding of how vaccines are developed, however, it's important to see how the vaccines produce an immune response, their 'mechanism of action', and how us humans develop the needed antibodies.

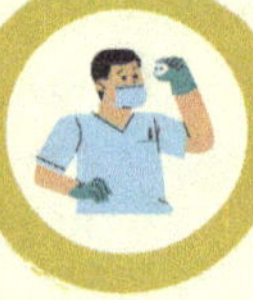

Understanding COVID-19 vaccines

How do the vaccines work?

MODERNA NIAID, AND PFIZER BIONTECH COVID-19 VACCINE

These are messenger RNA (mRNA) vaccines which essentially teach our cells how to make a protein that will trigger an immune response inside our bodies.

The mRNA is derived from the SARS-CoV-2 virus. Particularly from the S-protein by working backwards to find the mRNA that is being translated for the S-protein.

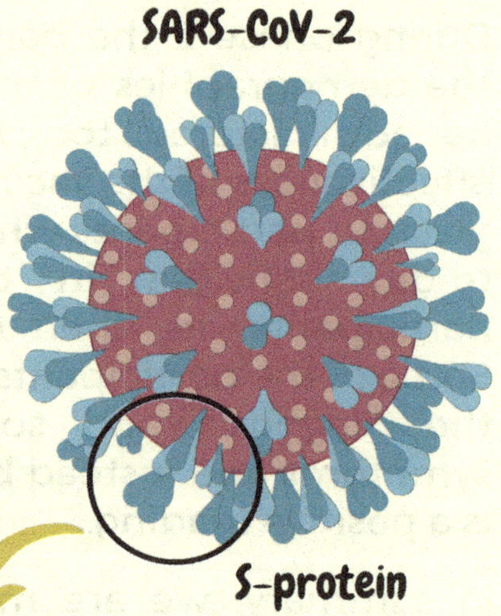

This mRNA is then wrapped with a lipid nanoparticle, which is just a phospholipid bilayer. This acts as a vehicle to transport the virus into the host cell.

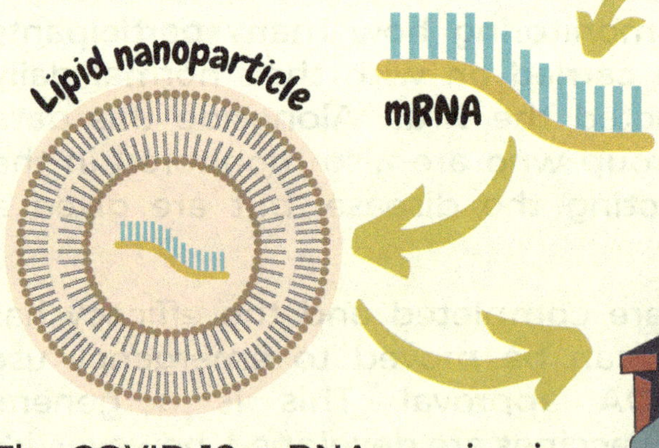

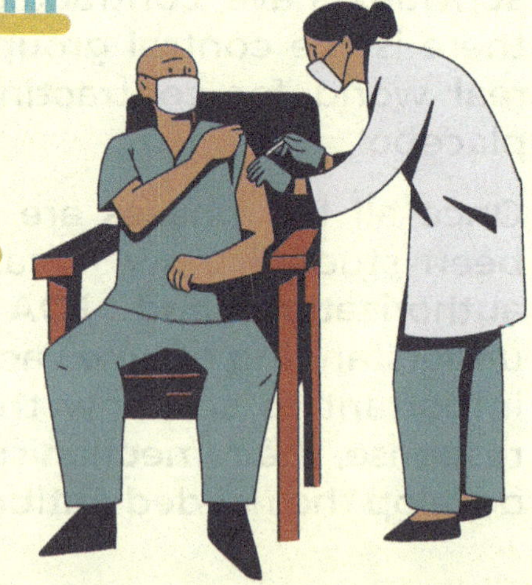

The COVID-19 mRNA vaccine is then injected into the upper arm muscle.

Mechanism of action MODERNA NIAID, AND PFIZER BIONTECH

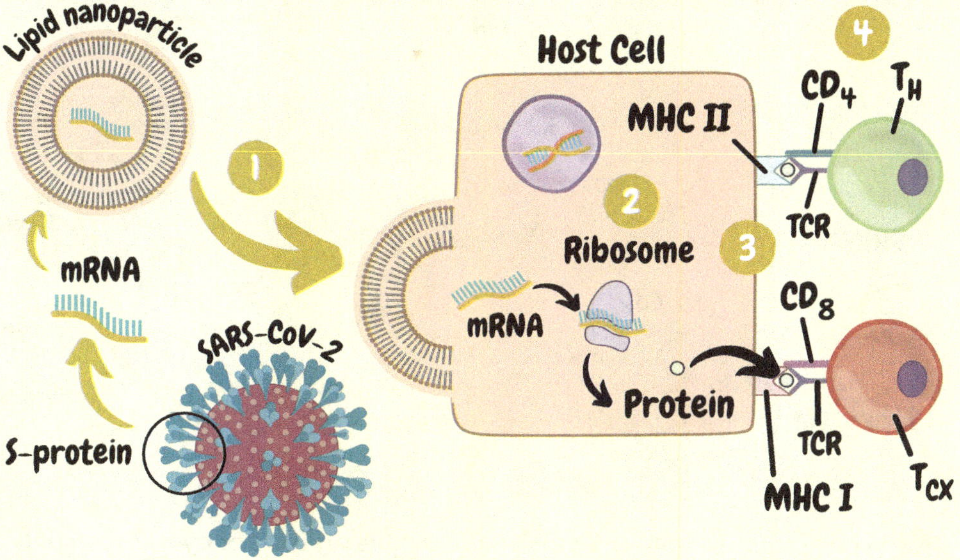

1. Lipid nano particle will fuse with a 'host cell' of the body and release the mRNA to enter the host cell.

2. Once the mRNA is inside it instructs and uses the cells' machinery, such as the ribosomes, for the process of 'translation'. This process uses the mRNA to create S-proteins.

3. The S-proteins are then expressed on the host cell's membrane onto two types of other proteins: MHC II complex proteins which are only found on antigen presenting cells such as B-cells (lymphocytes), macrophages, and dendritic cells. And the MHC I complex proteins, which are found on any cell that contains a nucleus. When the viral S-protein is expressed on the MHC I & II complexes it starts attracting our bodies immune cells.

EXPRESSION ON THE MHC II

4. Here comes the helper T cell (T_H) which on its membrane is equipped with two particular proteins: A TCR that interacts with the viral S-protein that is being presented and the CD4 that interacts directly with the MHC II protein. This interaction activates the helper T cell.

Understanding COVID-19 vaccines

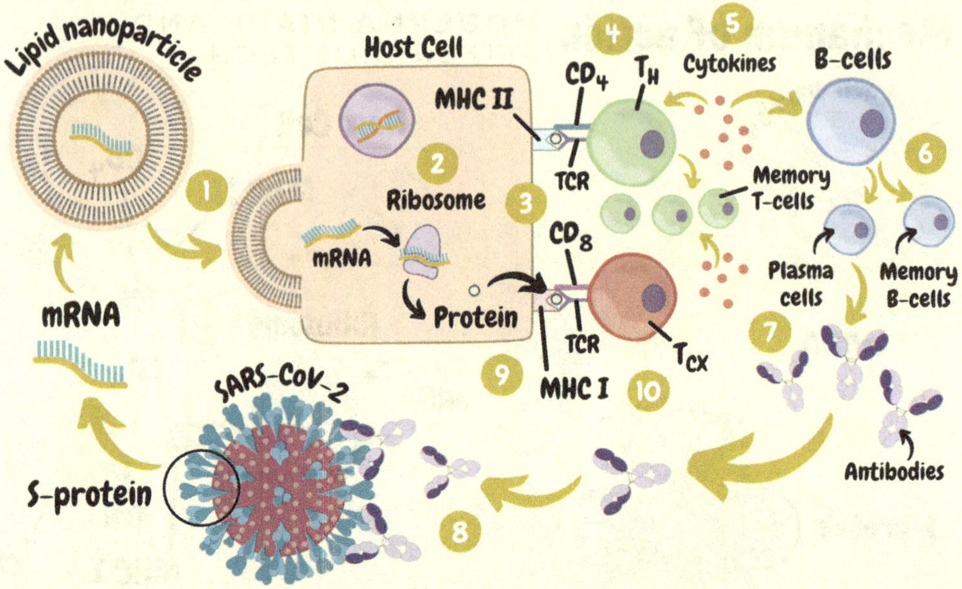

5 The activated helper T cell begins releasing tons of cytokines, such as interleukins (IL-2, IL-4, IL-5).

6 Cytokines tell the B-cells to start proliferating and differentiate into specialized cells called plasma cells and memory B-cells. The cytokines also stimulate the helper T cells to proliferate and differentiate to create memory T cells and effector T cells.

7 The plasma cells now begin creating antibodies which are specifically directed to go against the virus' S-proteins.

8 This antibody that binds to the virus can help neutralize the virus or enhance its destruction.

EXPRESSION ON THE MHC I

9 Along with the helper T cell, there is the cytotoxic T cell (T_{CX}) which is equipped with its TCR protein to interact with the MHC I. The cytotoxic T cell is different because it has a protein called the CD8 that attaches to the MHC I. The cytotoxic T cells also release cytokines that will amplify the 'MHC II - helper T cell process'.

10 The cytotoxic T cells release destructive molecules that destroy cells infected with the virus in the future.

Understanding COVID-19 vaccines

OXFORD/ASTRAZENECA COVID-19 VACCINE

The goal is the same, to create an antibody response to the S-protein found on the SARS-CoV-2 virus.

This vaccine uses a chimpanzee adenovirus which houses a DNA molecule. This DNA is essentially created by working backwards from the S-protein of SARS-CoV-2 to mRNA and then converting the mRNA to DNA. This DNA is now incorporated into the chimpanzee adenovirus.

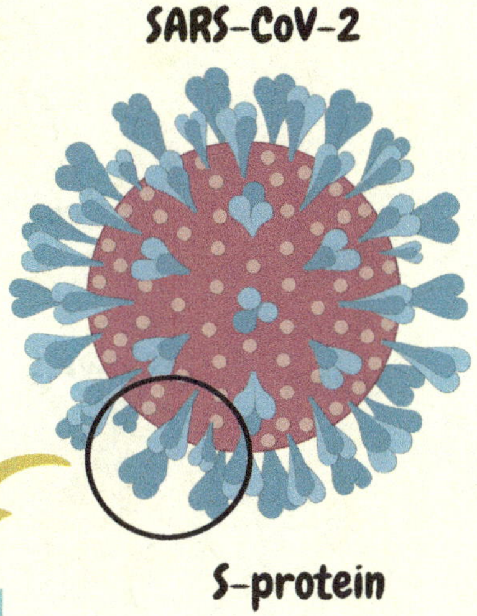

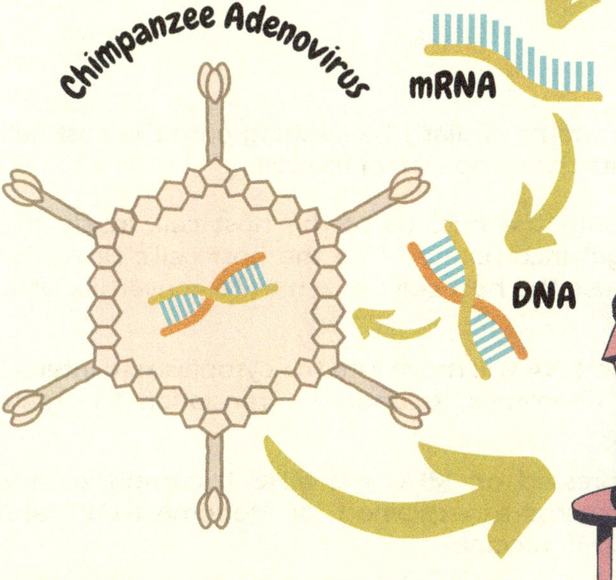

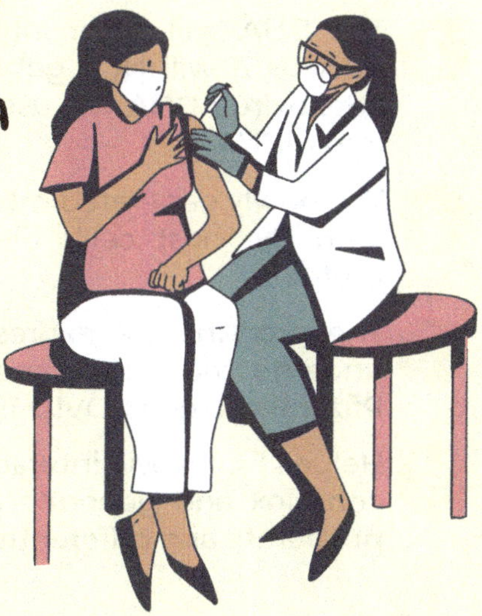

The COVID-19 vaccine can now be injected into the upper arm muscle.

Mechanism of action OXFORD/ASTRAZENECA

Chimpanzee adenovirus

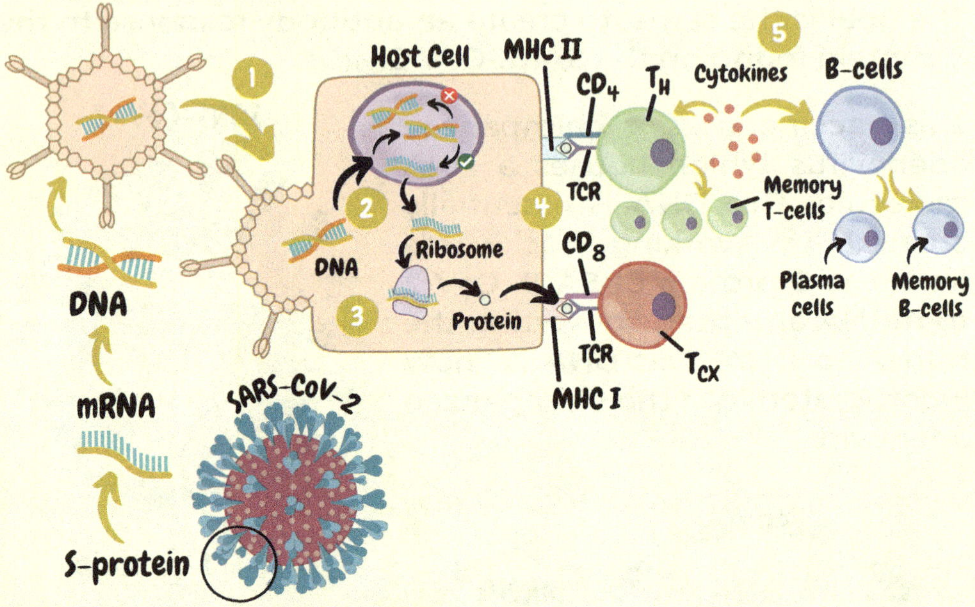

1. This adenovirus will perform similarly by latching onto the host cell and release its DNA into the cytoplasm of the cell.

2. The DNA will enter into the nucleus of the host cell. Inside the nucleus it will NOT get incorporated into the host cell's DNA. The adenovirus' DNA will use the host cell's enzymes to convert its DNA into mRNA.

3. The newly generated mRNA will move into the cytoplasm to interact with the host cell's ribosomes to undergo translation to create proteins.

4. The proteins are expressed on MHC I & MHC II complexes and undergo the same process as explained for Moderna NIAID, and Pfizer BioNTech COVID-19 vaccine.

5. Helper T cells will interact with the expressed protein on the MHC I complex and generate an immune response. This tells B-cells to proliferate and differentiate into plasma cells and memory B-cells.

Understanding COVID-19 vaccines

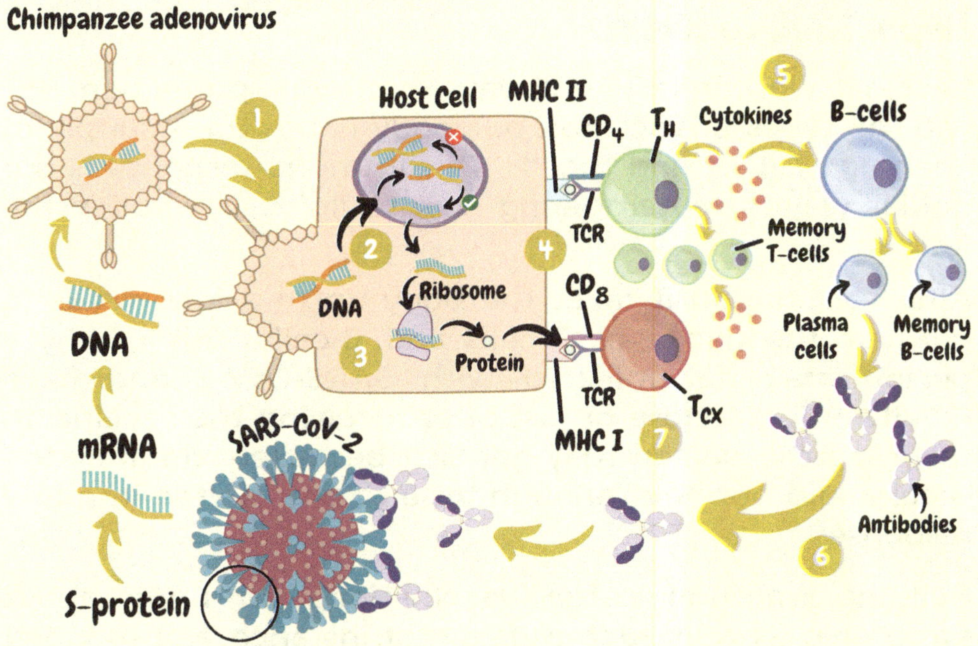

6 The plasma cells generate antibodies that will go after the S-protein on the SARS-CoV-2 virus.

7 The MHC II complex will also undergo the same process as before by expressing the protein for cytotoxic T cells to latch onto. These cytotoxic T cells will produce destructive molecules that will destroy the future cells infected with SARS-CoV-2 virus. Cytotoxic T cells will also release cytokines that will aid in the antibody response.

The body keeps a few T-cells, called "memory T cells," that go into action quickly if the body comes across the same virus again. When familiar foreign bodies are detected, B-cells produce antibodies to attack them. Researchers are still learning how long these memory cells protect a person against SARS-CoV-2 that causes COVID-19.

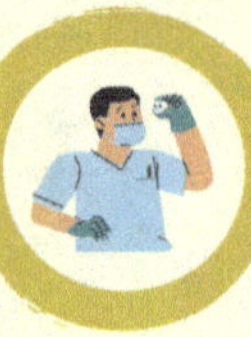

Understanding COVID-19 vaccines

Important to know

Vaccines work in different ways to provide protection. But with all types of vaccines, our body issues for a supply of 'memory' T-cells and B-cells. This immune response is our bodies way of remembering how to fight the virus in the future.

After vaccination it takes the body up to a few weeks to produce the necessary T-cells and B-cells. This is why a person may get infected with SARS-CoV-2 and have COVID-19 just before or just after receiving the vaccine. In this case the person may get sick because ultimately the vaccine did not have enough time to provide the immune response.

Building immunity after vaccination can bring about symptoms as well, such as fever for instance. Not to worry because these symptoms are normal and actually provides a great sign that our immunity is building.

In the case for Pfizer BioNTech and Moderna COVID-19 vaccines you are considered vaccinated when you receive two shots. And by two weeks after your second shot you will be considered fully vaccinated.

There are vaccines that require one shot, such as Johnson & Johnson's Janssen COVID-19 vaccine. It will also take up to two weeks after your shot to be considered fully vaccinated.

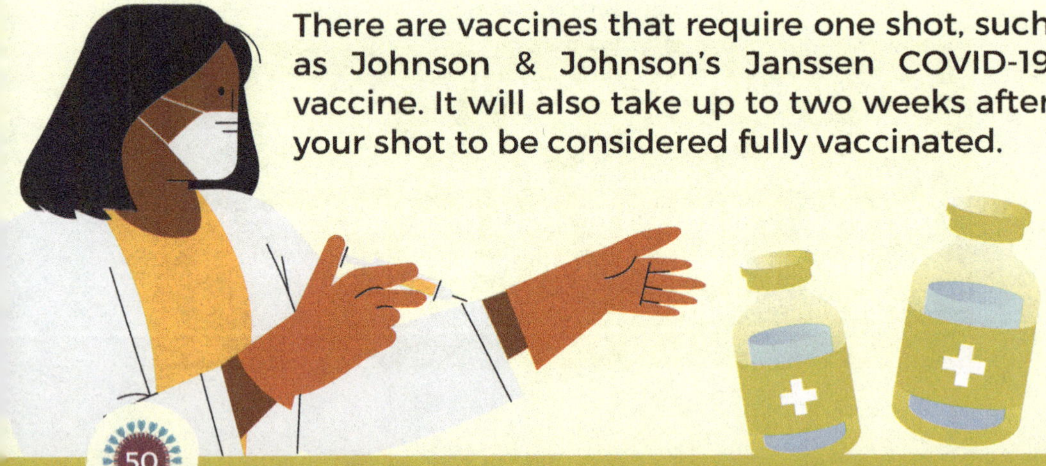

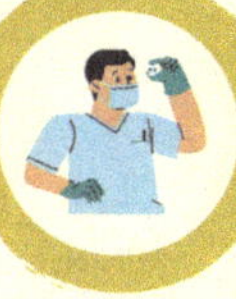

Booster Shots and Additional Doses

A booster shot is an additional dose of the vaccine given after the protection by the original vaccine series has begun to decrease over time. Booster is essentially designed so the vaccinated individual can maintain his or her immunity for longer. Anyone who is fully vaccinated and 16 years and older can get a booster.

An additional dose is given to individuals who are moderately to severely immunocompromised or who haven't built enough protection from their original vaccine. It is administered to these individuals in efforts to improve the response from their original vaccination. This appears to be the case for some immunocompromised people who received Pfizer-BioNTech or Moderna COVID-19 vaccines.

WHO IS MODERATELY OR SEVERELY IMMUNOCOMPROMISED?

- Receiving active cancer treatment for tumors or cancers of the blood
- Received an organ transplant and are taking medicine to suppress the immune system
- Received a stem cell transplant within the last 2 years or are taking medicine to suppress the immune system
- Moderate or severe primary immunodeficiency (such as DiGeorge syndrome, Wiskott-Aldrich syndrome)
- Advanced or untreated HIV infection
- Active treatment with high-dose corticosteroids or other drugs that may suppress your immune response

Please speak with your healthcare provider about your medical condition, and whether getting an additional primary shot is appropriate for you.

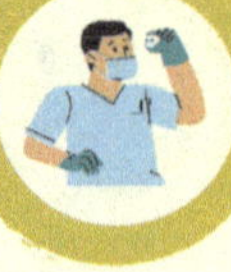

Understanding COVID-19 vaccines

Currently, moderately or severely immunocompromised people ages 18 years and older who completed their Moderna vaccine primary series should plan to get an additional primary dose 28 days after receiving their second shot. People ages 12 years and older who completed their Pfizer-BioNTech vaccine primary series should also plan to get an additional primary dose 28 days after receiving their second shot.

BOOSTER DOES NOT HAVE TO BE THE SAME BRAND.

You can mix and match brands. The FDA has authorized three vaccine boosters — Pfizer BioNTech, Moderna and Johnson & Johnson's Janssen — and determined that it is safe to get a COVID-19 vaccine booster or additional dose that is a different brand than your initial dose or doses. The Pfizer-BioNTech vaccine is the only vaccine and booster authorized for individuals ages 16 and 17.

If you get the Moderna booster, you will receive half of the original Moderna dose. Please be sure to confirm this with the person giving you the shot.

Even highly effective vaccines often become less effective over time, and the coronavirus vaccines are no exception. Initial evidence on mRNA vaccines like Pfizer and Moderna suggest they start to lose some of their power against infection and serious illness, regardless of variant of the virus.

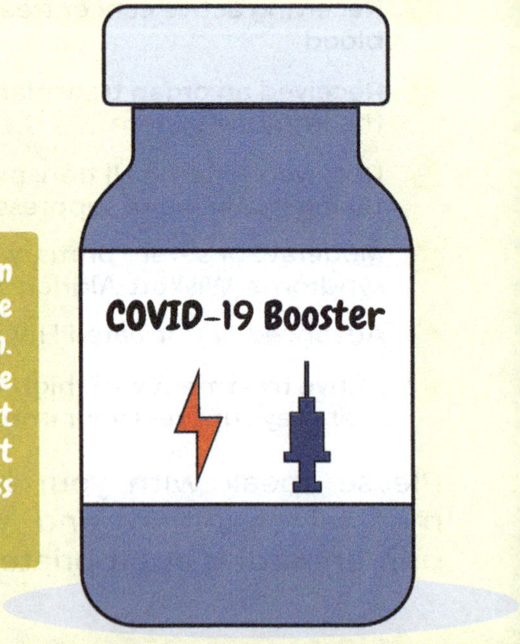

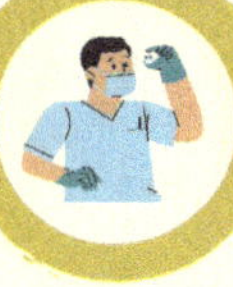

Self-Care

If you have mild symptoms, try to stay at home until you have recovered. Here is a quick way to relieve your symptoms:

Fever

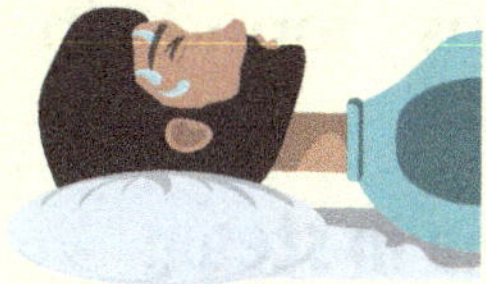

The average body temperature is 98.6°F (37°C) and the 'normal' temperature varies from person to person.

A fever is a sign that our body is trying to fight an illness or infection. It is identified with a temperature reading of 100.4°F (38°C) or higher.

Over the counter medication

You can take ibuprofen, naproxen, acetaminophen or aspirin. It can help relieve head and body aches and lower your temperature.

Get Rest!

Your body needs the rest and helps your body build up its immune response.

Drink plenty of fluids

Stay hydrated as fevers often cause sweating - loss of water from the body. Have water or juice and stay away from soda or any high sugar beverages (which actually make you thirstier).

Shortness of Breath

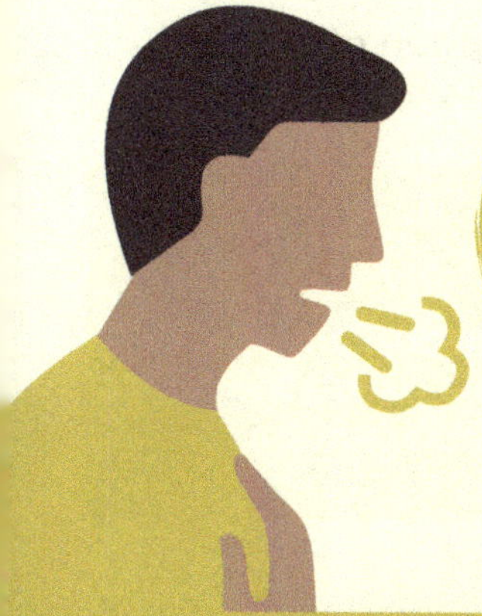

Relax and breathe slower

Improve your breathing by taking slower breaths. Pair this with mindfulness and meditation techniques to attain a more calm and peaceful state of mind. You will not only breathe better but also relieve any anxiety, which could be causing the shortness of breath.

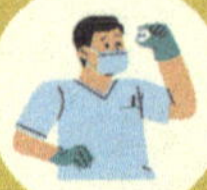

Cough

Stay hydrated and drink warm beverages

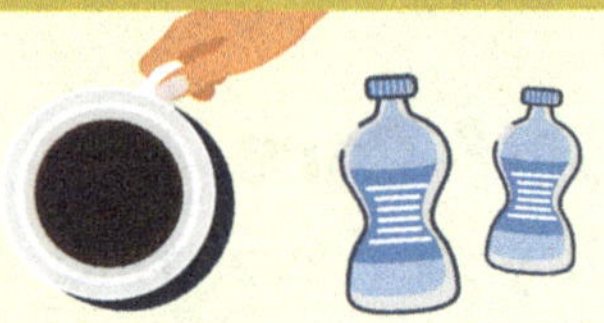

Keeping the throat moist is key to ease a cough. Having warm beverages can help break up mucus found in the upper airways and throat.

Have honey with tea or hot water

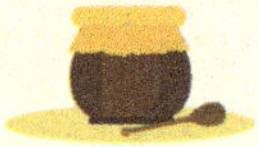

A drop of honey is a well-tested way to soothe a sore throat and can even be an effective cough suppressant.

Breathe in steam

Try using a humidifier, vaporizer or simply taking a hot shower. Moisture produced in the air while showering can help ease coughing, moisten the throat and help reduce pain and scratchiness.

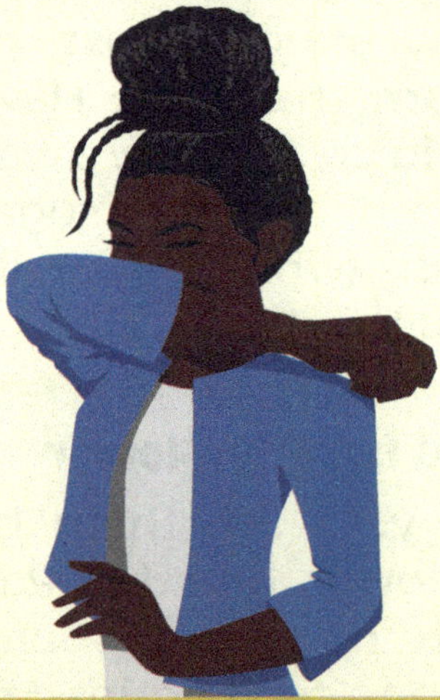

You can also try

- Cough drops and lozenges

- Cough medicine:
  For a wet cough with mucus you should take something that will get the mucus out.
  For a dry cough take a cough suppressant.

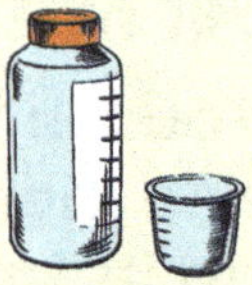

- Gargle salt water: 1 teaspoon of salt in 8 ounces of warm water.

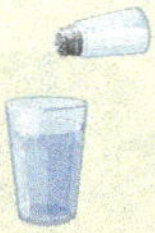

Notice the coughing etiquette!

Cough or sneeze into the fold of your arm. This ensures the germs are not on your hands. Or use a tissue that you throw away immediately in a plastic-lined wastebasket.

Recover at home safe

Most individuals will have mild symptoms and there are many easy ways to ease the symptoms. After a few days of feeling symptoms, majority of individuals start feeling better and some will have a sense of being completely fine within a week. However, this is not a reason for the individual to step out in public or be amongst family members. The individual is still contagious and should remain in isolation for the complete 14 days from the start of symptoms.

Your body is fighting the virus, so let it do its job. Focus your attention on staying away from other people, practicing good hand washing, hygiene and cleanliness protocols. By doing all this, you will be sure to have protected your loved ones from contracting the virus.

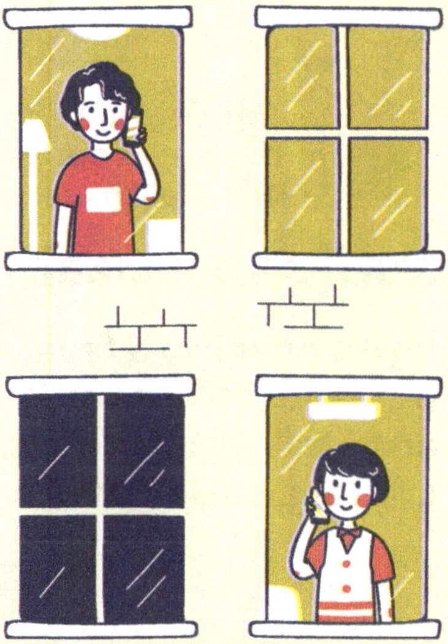

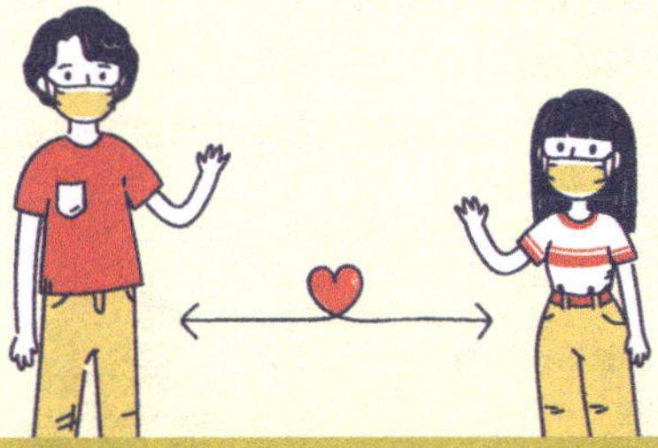

Be gentle with yourself and stay calm

You and others around you may experience difficult times dealing with COVID-19, and it is thus crucial to remain calm. You can try techniques like mindfulness, breathing exercises, and meditation to find your happy medium.

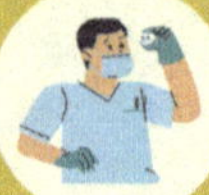

Treatment in a Hospital

For standard symptoms of COVID-19, such as mild fever and cough, there is no need to go to the hospital or ER. Hospitals will send you home if the symptoms can be treated at home with self-care. If you are feeling severely ill, the hospital staff will check for indications which can result in a more severe issue. They could do the following:

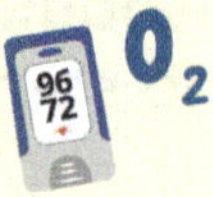

Check the oxygen levels in the blood with a finger clip monitor.

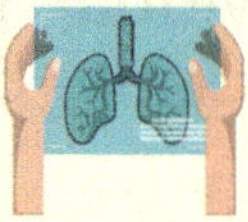

Listen to the lungs and monitor your breathing or perform a chest X-ray and CT scan.

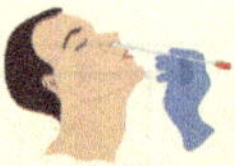

Administer a COVID-19 test.

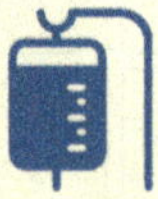

Administer IV fluids through your arm to prevent dehydration. In serious cases, they will connect you to a ventilator, which will breathe for you.

Notify your healthcare provider

If you develop a fever, cough, and difficulty breathing, reach out and seek medical care immediately. Call in advance, and tell your healthcare provider of any recent travel, contact, or dealings with anyone who has the disease.

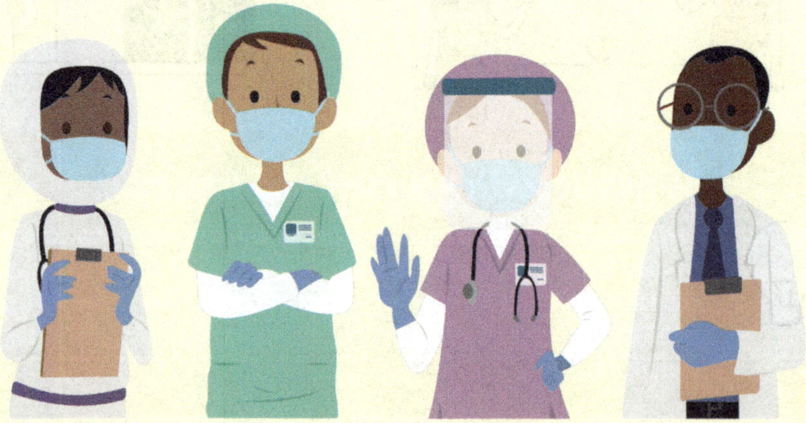

7 How does COVID-19 spread?

- Person to person contact
- Viruses on surfaces
- Getting tested
  - Molecular Tests
  - Serological Tests

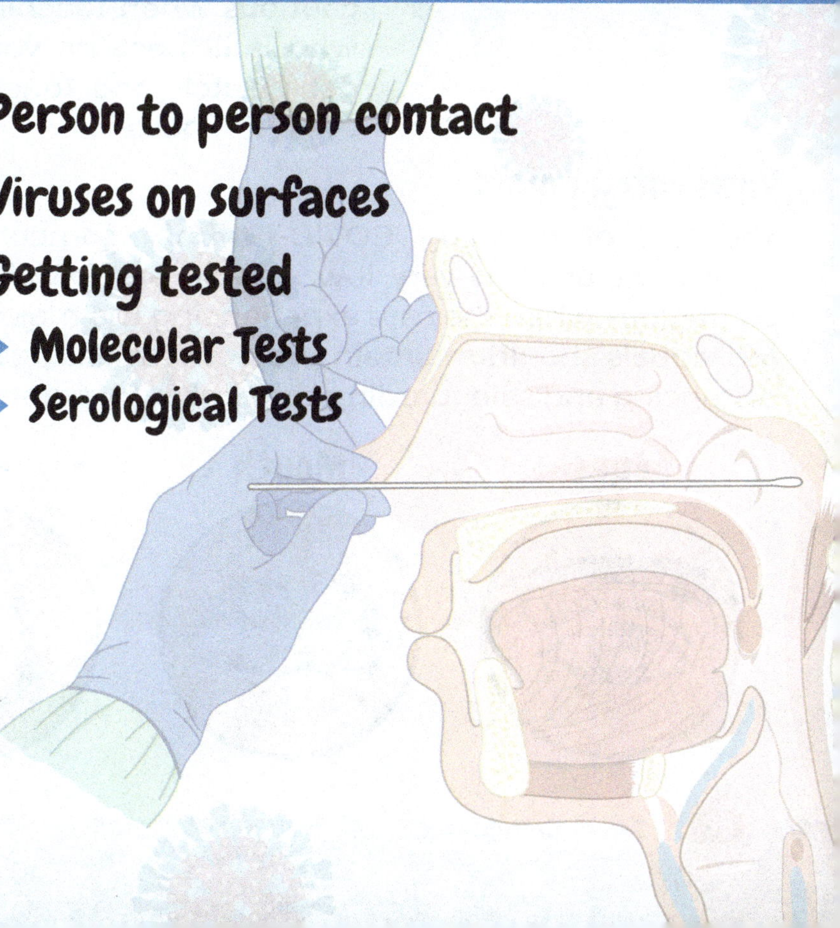

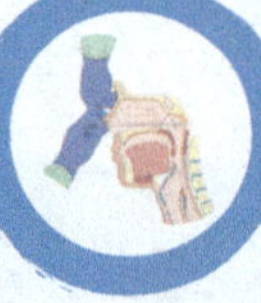

How does COVID-19 spread?

Person to person contact

Individuals are at high risk of contracting the virus when a person is in close contact (within 6 feet) with someone who has respiratory symptoms (e.g. coughing or sneezing). It is thus recommended to always maintain at least a distance of about 2 arms' length from someone who is sick.

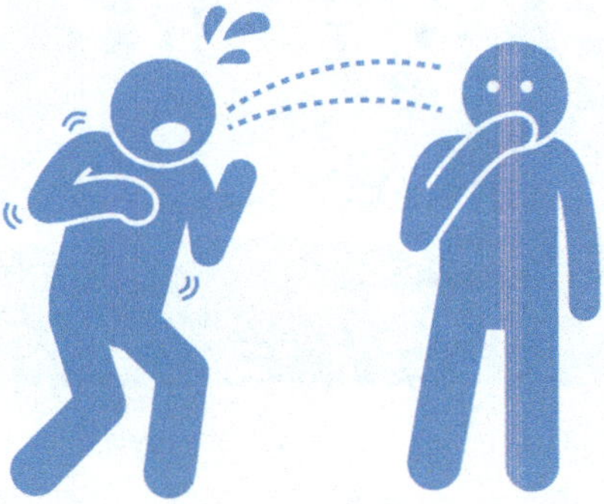

Its main way of spreading is droplet infection. The sites of entry of SARS-CoV-2 are the eyes, mouth, and nose. When people cough or sneeze, the droplets can land in the mouths or noses of others. It is important to be cautious when touching someone who is ill because you can easily get an itch and touch your face, eyes, and nose.

Viral entry points

The risk of catching COVID-19 from someone with no symptoms at all is very low. People are found to be most contagious when they are experiencing the major symptoms. Individuals should maintain protective measures by physical distancing and safeguarding the viral entry points.

Eyes

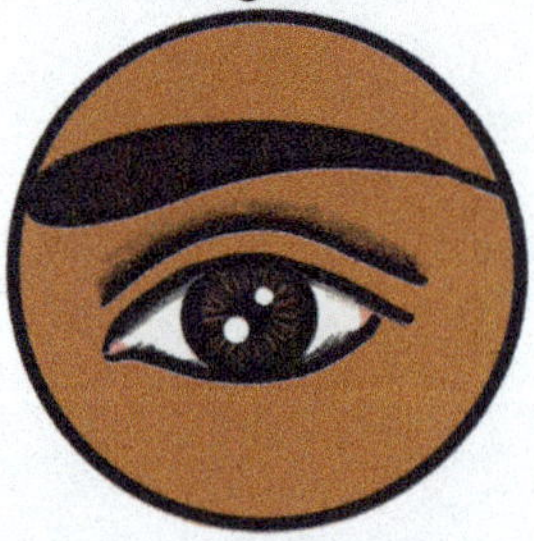

Mouth

Nose

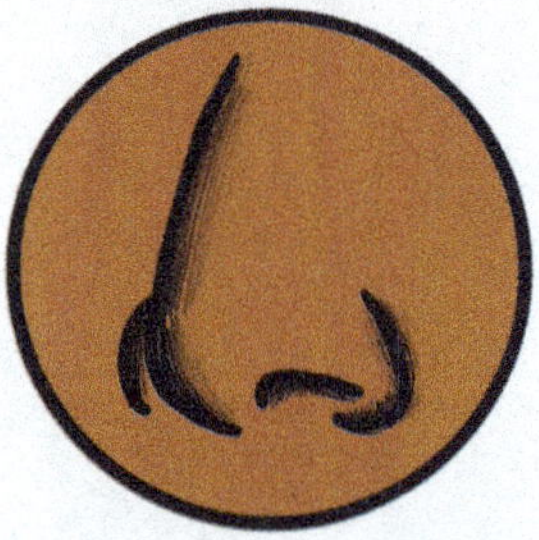

How does COVID-19 spread?

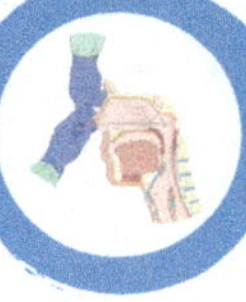

Viruses on surfaces

COVID-19 may spread via surfaces, but it is still uncertain how long it can survive on them. There are also reports indicating that COVID-19 can be transmitted through the air and from feces of someone with the disease. Air transmission is being argued, and there is a rather low chance of catching it via feces from an infected person.

Studies have provided suggestions on how long it can last outside the body on surfaces:

As aerosol in the air →	Up to 3 hours
On copper →	Up to 4 hours
On cardboard →	Up to 24 hours
On plastic and stainless steel →	2-3 days
On wood and glass →	5 days

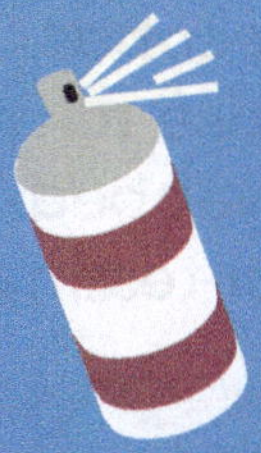

Aerosol

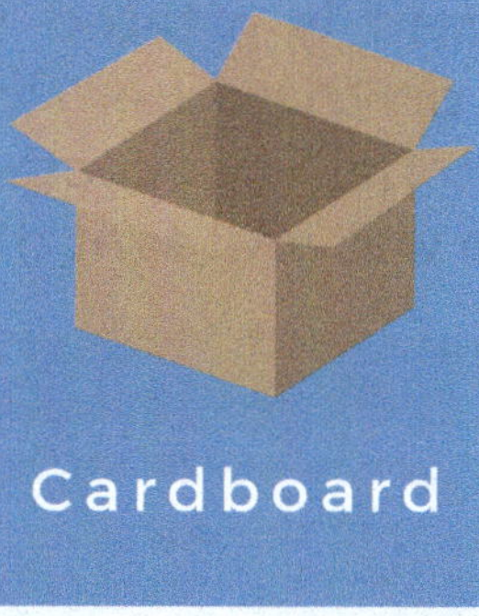

Cardboard

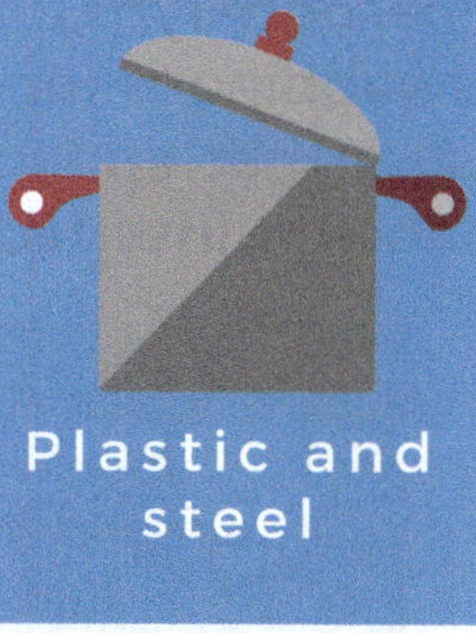

Plastic and steel

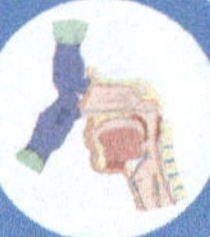

How does COVID-19 spread?

There are two main types of tests for COVID-19, namely, molecular and serological. Molecular testing refers to tests that detect if we currently have the virus, and serological testing refers to tests that detect if we currently have antibodies to that virus. Both categories of testing are important to understand who is infected and the possibility of transmission of the virus.

There is ongoing research to test those who had the virus and are immune – these individuals might be able to help others with treatment possibilities.

Getting tested

SCIENCE INVOLVED IN MOLECULAR TESTING

When an individual has signs and symptoms of COVID-19, the genetic material from the virus SARS-CoV-2 is detectable in the upper and lower parts of the respiratory tract. In less severe infections, molecular tests are used to detect the presence of the virus in a collected sample.

We are not used to people sticking long plastic sticks inside our nose, and it can be a little uncomfortable. The tissues in the area are sensitive to touch, which can result in a sneeze, or a runny nose. The 6-inch-long swab travels into the nasal cavity to reach the area between the nose and mouth (nasopharynx). The swab is rotated for 10-15 seconds, and swabbing is repeated on the other side of the nose to make sure that enough material is collected. Once swabbed, it is labeled, inserted into a vial, and sent off to a lab for testing.

The procedure is also commonly used to evaluate individuals with suspected respiratory infection caused by other viruses and bacteria.

Molecular Tests

NASOPHARYNGEAL SWAB TECHNIQUE

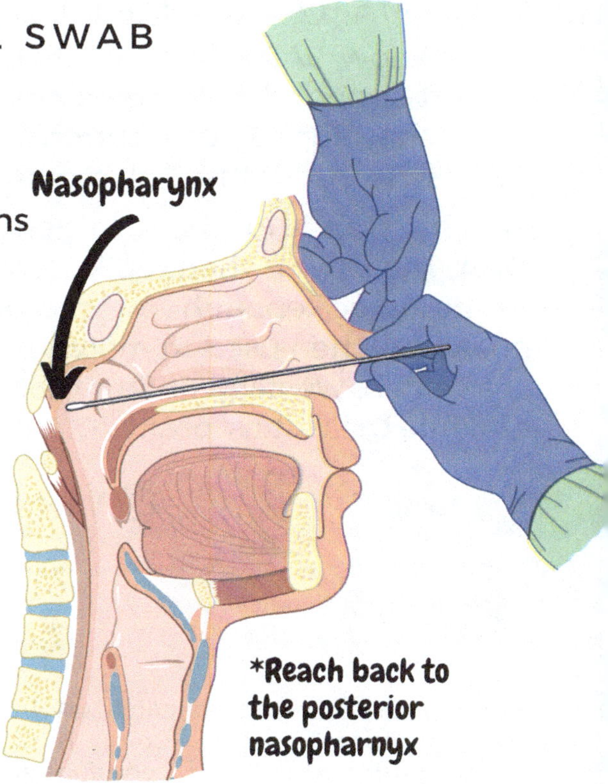

1. Have patient blow nose into a tissue to clear excess secretions
2. Instruct patient to tilt the head slightly and close their eyes to lessen the mild discomfort of the procedure
3. Gently insert the swab along the nasal septum just above the floor of the nasal cavity
4. Reach for the nasopharynx until resistance is felt
5. Rotate the swab against the nasopharyngeal mucosa for 10-15 seconds
6. Gently remove the swab and place it into its container

Be thoughtful!

As you notice symptoms begin to progress, pick up the phone and call your healthcare provider, and tell them about your exposure and symptoms. The healthcare provider will be better able to access you and advise whether to get tested.

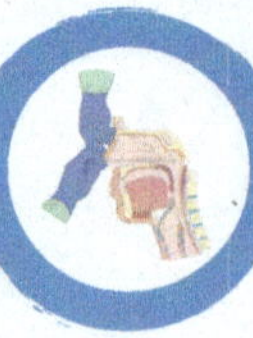

How does COVID-19 spread?

RT-PCR: REVERSE TRANSCRIPTASE POLYMERASE CHAIN REACTION

As we know, SARS-CoV-2 contains a genetic code made up of a short-stranded RNA sequence. While new techniques are being developed, the current method in the lab is the Reverse Transcriptase Polymerase Chain Reaction (RT-PCR).

The first step is for the RNA genetic code to be converted to DNA. The DNA is then replicated in order for the sample size to be large enough for thorough genetic analysis. This analysis is then used to match the profile of the virus. If there is a match, we can confirm that there is indeed an infection, and rule the test as 'positive'.

1 Swab

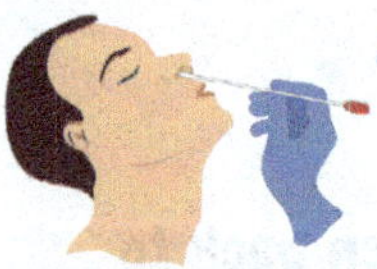

Samples are collected from the patient's nose or throat using a swab. The sample is sent to a lab.

2 Viral ssRNA

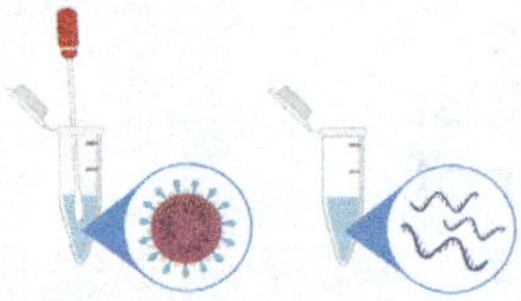

Viral ssRNA of SARS-CoV-2 is extracted by centrifuge and chemical reagents.

3 The Mix

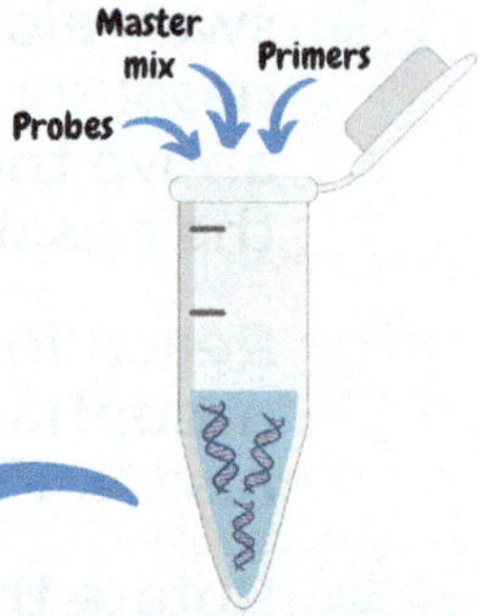

Extracted RNA is added to a master mixture with primers and probes.

4 PCR machine

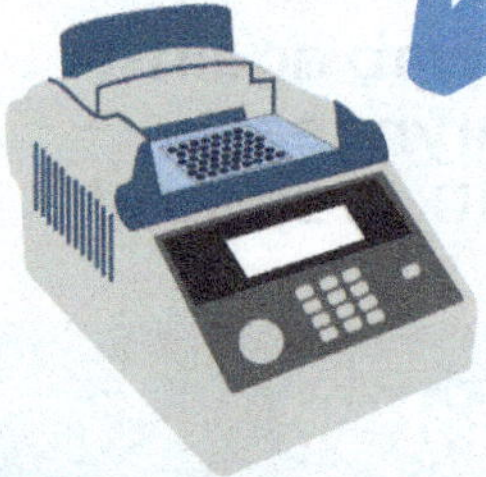

The tube is placed in a PCR machine, where it is converted into DNA, it is amplified, and fluorescence is attached. The amount of double-stranded DNA is doubled in each cycle of the machine.

5 Analysis

With the measurement of the fluorescent signal, real-time data is collected.

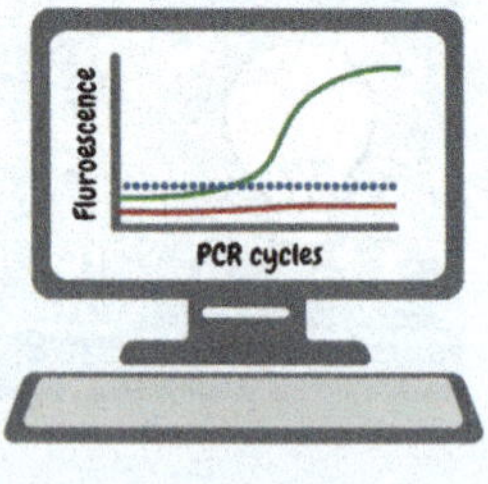

Results

Positive

When there is viral genetic material in the sample, amplification occurs, releasing enough fluorescent markers to be detected.

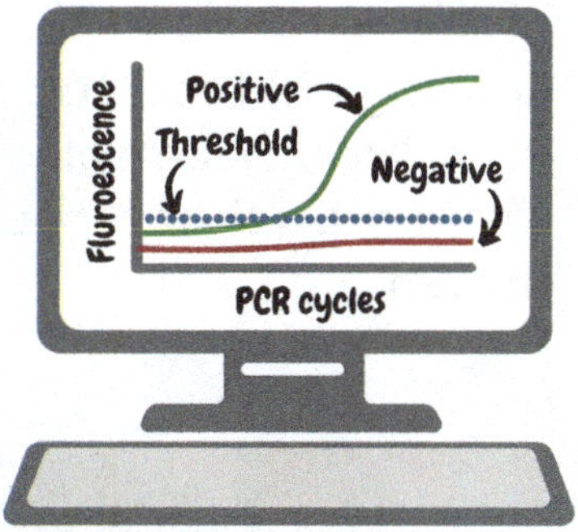

Negative

If there is **no** viral genetic material in the sample, amplification **does not occur**, and no fluorescent markers are detected.

How quickly can we expect results?

Most RT-PCR tests take a few hours, or up to 3-4 days, but lab companies are working diligently to provide at-home or quicker alternatives to testing.

How accurate is molecular testing?

While the positive test indicates an active viral SARS-CoV-2 particle and COVID-19 infection, it does not rule out other bacterial or viral co-infections. There is also a possibility for the test to be **false positive**, and the patient does not have the COVID-19 infection.

A result which is negative means that the virus that is causing COVID-19 was not detected in the sample above the limit of detection. However, there is still a possibility for very low levels of the virus in our body even after testing negative.

False negatives are possible, and these should be considered if there are any apparent signs and symptoms of COVID-19, travel history, or exposure to those with the infection.

It is thus advisable for individuals to follow up with a second testing method, that is, the serological method, in order to test for antibodies.

Serological Tests (Antibodies)

SCIENCE INVOLVED IN SEROLOGICAL TESTING

Serological tests focus on detecting antibodies in a blood sample, which is obtained by a simple prick of the finger or having blood drawn.

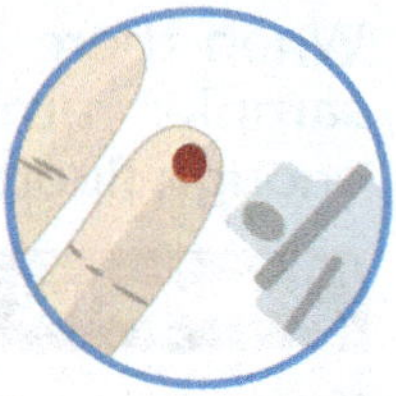

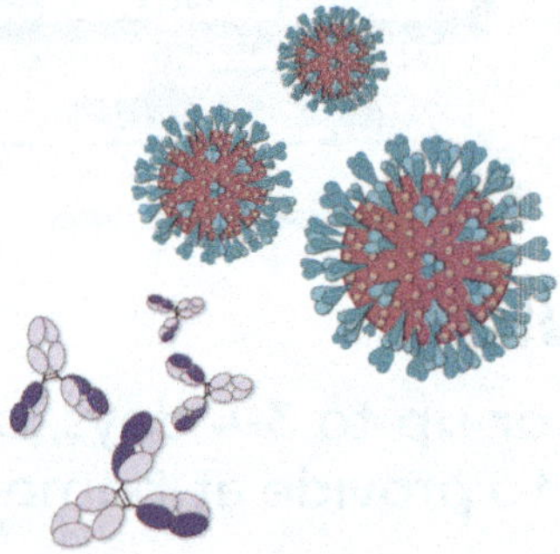

Antibodies are special protein molecules that our immune system produces in response to foreign particles (antigens). A virus entering our body is a great example of an antigen, and one way our body's immune system responds is by producing antibodies, which bond to the SARS-CoV-2 particle and work to neutralize it.

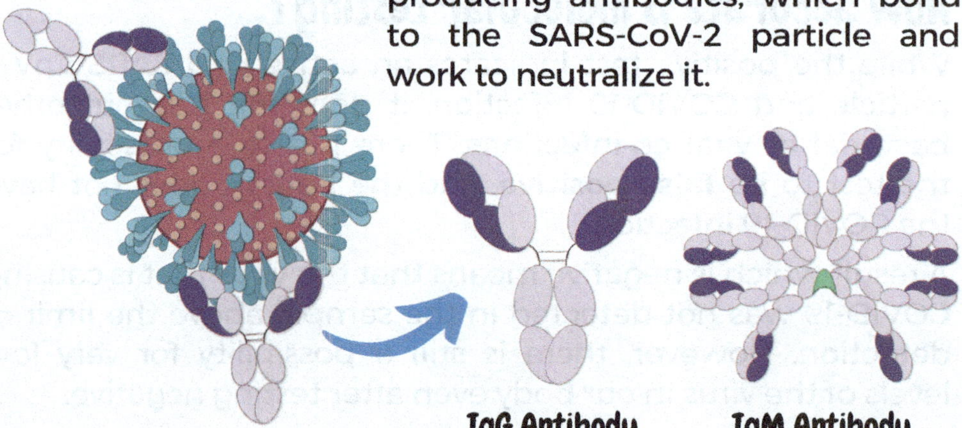

Testing for antibodies looks for the presence of IgM antibodies, which appear early in an infection, and indicate recent exposure to COVID-19. It further looks for IgG antibodies, which remain in the blood, and provide long-term protection even after we have recovered.

There is still much to learn about how strongly antibodies respond to new viruses like SARS-CoV-2, and how long any immune protection may persist. But there are investigations to see whether enough antibodies are present in an individual's blood, and whether it would be possible for healthcare providers to use the blood plasma to treat others.

Important to note!
An antibody test is not performed to check for the virus, but rather to see whether our immune system has responded to the infection. Additionally, current antibody tests do not tell us if we are in fact immune to COVID-19. This is because researchers don't know how long these antibodies protect us from the virus.

How quickly can we expect results?

Much faster than molecular tests. This is because these tests do not require special equipment and personnel to analyze the results. Turnaround time can be as quick as 1-2 days.

How accurate is serological testing?

Our body can take up to several days or even weeks to develop an immune response to the virus, such as, producing the antibodies. Therefore, serological tests may not be useful to detect the current infection, and thus, an individual may be led to think that they don't have the infection when they actually do.

But the good news is that these tests can identify individuals who have had the infection and since then recovered.

It is still not clear to medical professionals and researchers if being infected means that we cannot be infected again. The testing should not determine if we are immune to being re-infected.

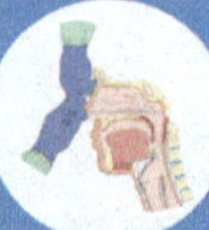

How does COVID-19 spread?

Priority list for getting tested

Priority 1

Healthcare facility workers with symptoms

Hospitalized patients

Priority 2

Patients in long-term care facilities with symptoms

Patients 65 years of age and older with symptoms

Patients with underlying conditions with symptoms

First responders with symptoms

Priority 3

Critical infrastructure workers with symptoms

Healthcare facility workers and first responders

Individuals with mild symptoms in communities experiencing high numbers of COVID-19 hospitalizations

Individuals who do not meet any of the above categories with symptoms

***For more info visit: coronavirus.gov**

Incubation period

The 'incubation period' is the time between catching the virus and beginning to have symptoms of the disease. Most estimates of the incubation period for COVID-19 range from 1-14 days, most commonly around five days. These estimates are updated as more data becomes available.

8 Understanding the New Normal

- Flattening the curve
- Leaving our homes
  - When is it safe?
  - Consider the risks
  - Practice every day preventative actions
- Social and Physical distancing
- Hand washing and Hygiene
- Quarantine

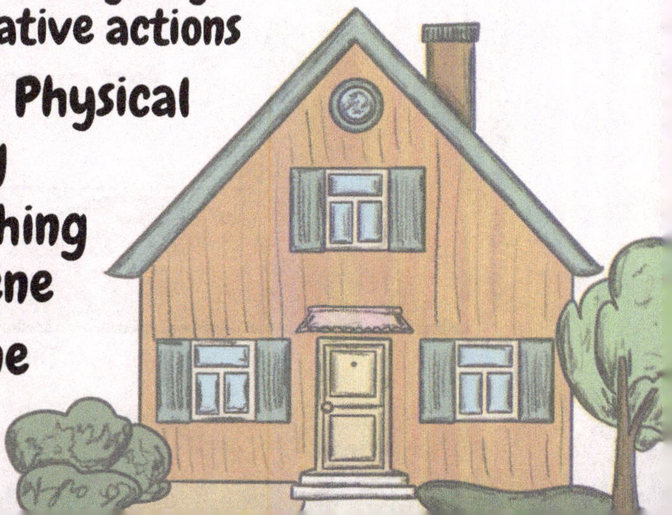

People across the world sheltered in their homes and apartments amidst the COVID-19 outbreak. With organizations, government leadership, and the unification of the general public, people quickly understood how physical and social distancing can 'flatten the curve', restrain the spread of the virus, and prevent the healthcare systems from failing. In essence, the alliance of communities and the protective measures that are in place are to target the virus only to 'buy more time', that is, the time needed to prepare for our next response.

The reality is that, until there is a vaccine developed to combat COVID-19, we will not return to life as we knew it. As long as people lack immunity, returning to normal carries the risk of potential infections. Therefore, as we step out of our safe places, we must understand the 'New Normal'. Planning, executing, and educating ourselves about COVID-19 and its safety measures is the best thing we can do.

Flattening the curve

The first phase in a pandemic response is containment. There are two ways how the crisis can go, namely, through a fast spread or a slow spread. The key is how the world manages it in its early days.

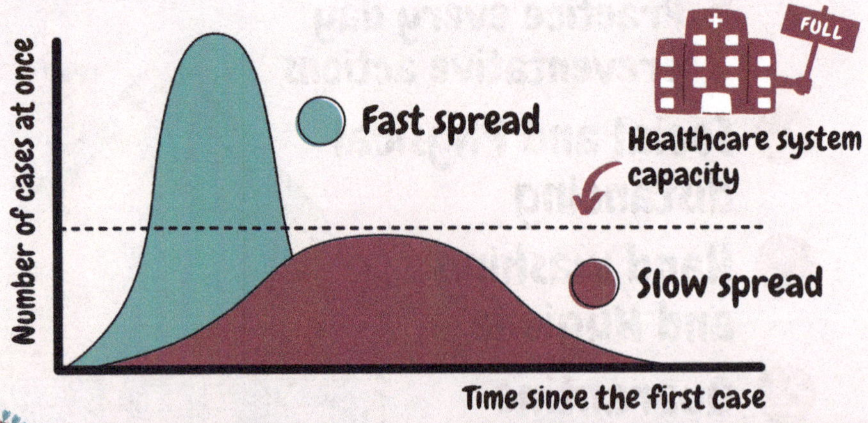

Fast spread can be destructive, and it is seen when many people are getting sick at the same time. Consequently, healthcare facilities reach their full capacities and become overwhelmed, not only because of those who have COVID-19, but also because other patients are admitted for heart attacks, trauma, seizures, strokes, and so forth. There is not enough equipment, staff, or ventilators for the influx of patients requiring them.

When a high number of people get sick, hospitals are forced to refuse people, who can even die untreated. This is a serious issue because, as healthcare staff get sick themselves, the foundations begin to crumble.

During this phase, it is necessary to enforce safety measures (e.g. social and physical distancing, sheltering, etc.) to limit the number of infections and ultimately give relief to healthcare systems. Therefore, when you start leaving your homes, remember to avoid **MEN**, and instead follow **WOMEN**.

AVOID MEN & FOLLOW WOMEN

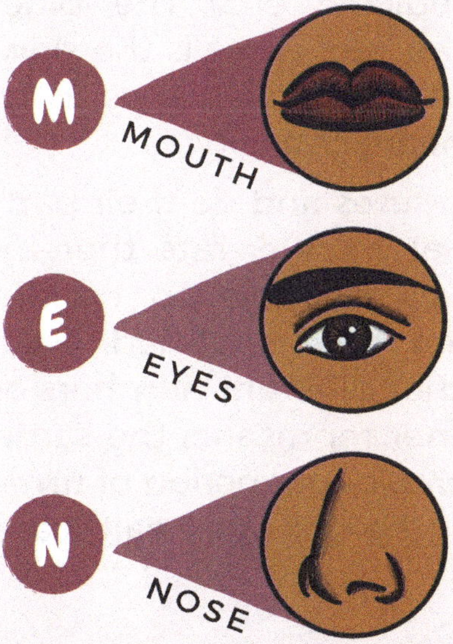

- **W** ash your hands with soap and water
- **O** bey social and physical distancing
- **M** ask on when outside home
- **E** xercise and eat well
- **N** o unnecessary traveling

TAKING A LOOK AT THE CURVE

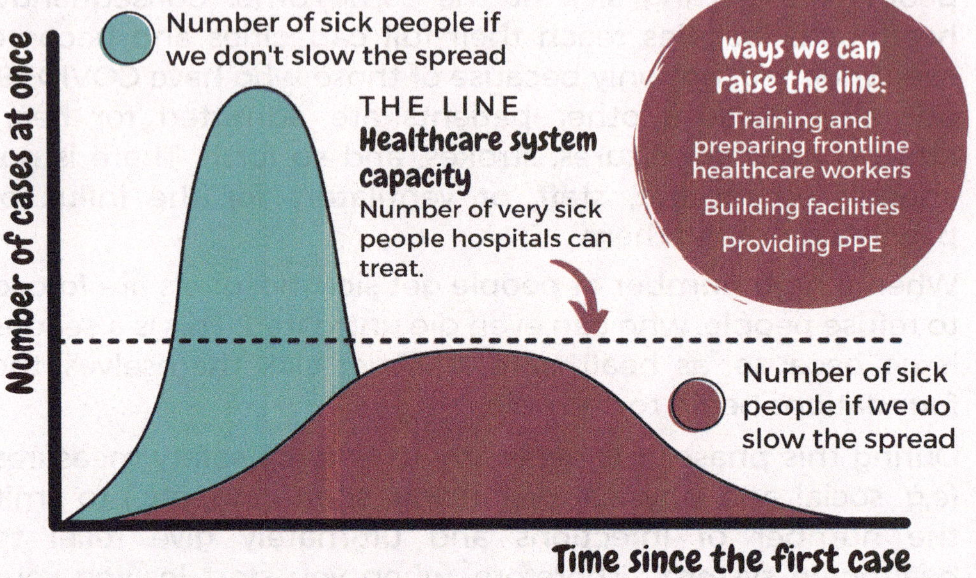

Labeled on the graph, we see a representation of the number of new COVID-19 cases since the onset of the disease. The dotted line is a measure of the healthcare system's capacity (i.e. staff, number of beds, PPE, medicine, etc.). The 'blue' curve represents a fast spread, and the 'red' curve is the slow spread. As we can see, flattening out the curve allows us to handle the pandemic with full healthcare capacity.

If people take serious protective measures and do their part, it ensures that individuals get sick at a lower rate thereby allowing the healthcare systems to be able to handle incoming sick patients without being overwhelmed. Note that the flatter curve doesn't mean that different numbers of people are being affected, but it rather represents the same number of people, but stretched over a longer period of time. Our goal is to raise the line by strengthening the healthcare system and flattening the curve.

3 ACTION ITEMS FOR A SAFE RETURN TO NORMALCY

1 Proper systems in place to track the virus

Communities at large must receive technology, resources, and constant alerts in order to track their health, medical cases, and deaths.

2 Modernize and supply hospital care systems

Hospitals and critical care clinics need better infrastructure to safely handle large numbers of patients. For example, staffing and room capacity must be able to handle outbreaks of disease, such as, COVID-19. It is also critical for the hospital staff to be equipped with ample amounts of personal protective equipment and measures in place to secure their safety.

3 Identify, test, and trace

As the world re-opens, millions of tests must be readily available to schools, businesses and facilities. Temperature screening are not sufficient to determine those who are infected with SARS-CoV-2. Other than identifying and testing infected individuals, there must be a method to trace their contacts, and isolate them from spreading the virus.

IDENTIFY

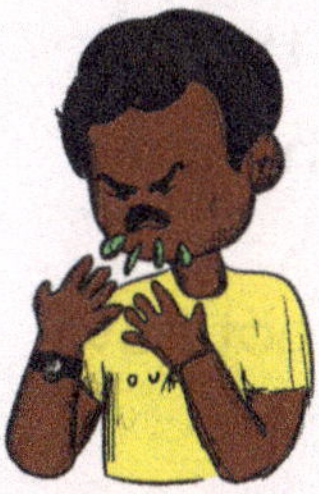

TEST

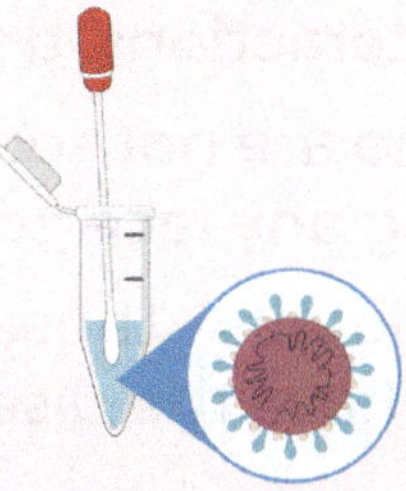

TRACE

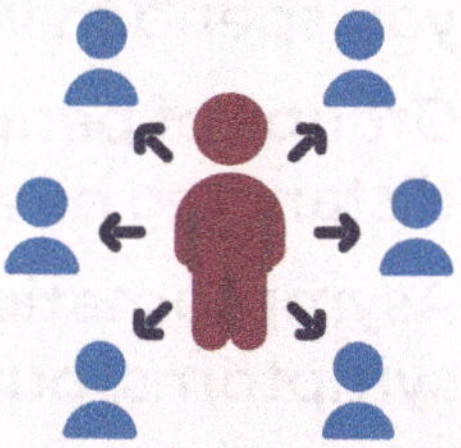

Leaving our homes

WHEN IS IT SAFE?

There is no way to ensure a zero risk of infection. But it is necessary to understand the risks and preventive protocols to follow in order to help reduce the spread of COVID-19.

If you have COVID-19, have symptoms that resemble those of COVID-19, or have been in close contact with someone who is ill with the disease, it is necessary for you to stay home and isolate yourself from others. When leaving your home, always have:

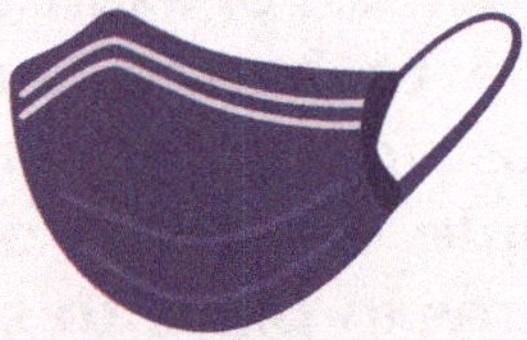

A mask or cloth face covering

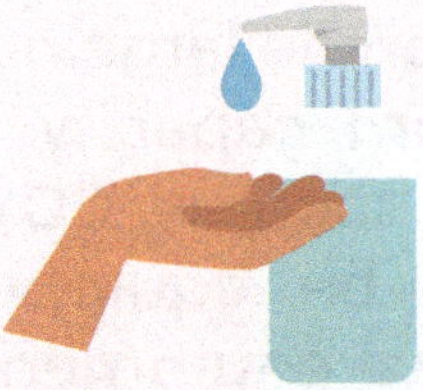

Hand sanitizer (at least 60% alcohol)

Important to note!

The more closely you interact with others, and the longer the duration of your interaction, the higher the risk of contracting and spreading the COVID-19 infection.

CONSIDER THE RISKS

- The more people you interact with, and the more time you spend in your interactions, the greater the risk.
- Groups of people who are not social and physical distancing or wearing any face covering.
- Asymptomatic individuals – those who do not have symptoms, but may have the disease.

- Is there at least 6 feet (2 meters) distance between you and those who you are with? The closer you are to those who may be infected, the greater the risk of falling ill.
- When using any type of transportation, follow respiratory etiquette when sneezing or coughing. Limit touching such surfaces as machines, handrails, restroom surfaces, benches, etc.
- Less ventilation and indoor spaces may put you at higher risk by being closer to those who may be infected. Outdoor spaces are hence recommended.
- Try to use touchless payment when dealing with transactions. Credit cards or cash can be placed in a receipt tray or on the counter when purchasing something.

PRACTICE PREVENTIVE ACTIONS

When leaving your home, be sure to review updates from your local health authorities in order to be current with stay-at-home orders, curfews, closures, and any breaking news. As we know, the SARS-CoV-2 particle travels when we are in close contact with someone who is ill; therefore, be sure to always practice social and physical distancing and wear face covering.

Continue to take extra precautions with the elderly and those with underlying medical conditions, especially if you live with someone who is at risk. These individuals have a higher risk of severe illness from COVID-19, and must be carefully handled. Keep practicing preventive actions, such as, monitoring your symptoms, not touching your face with unwashed hands, practicing good hygiene, and disinfecting surfaces.

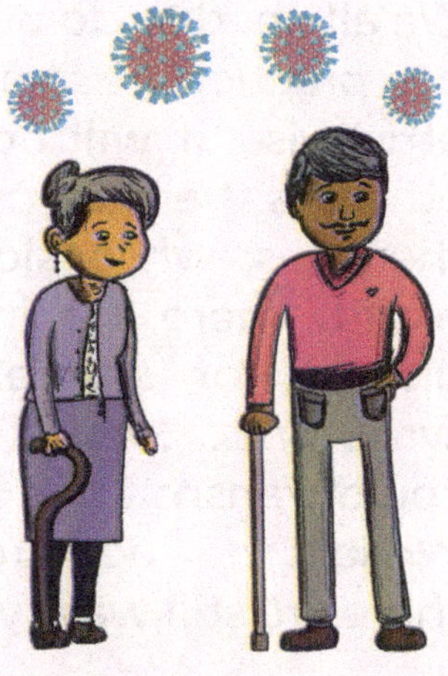

Social and Physical distancing

Helps keep vulnerable people safe. Think about your grandma, or someone else's grandma! One of the best things we can all do to stop the spread of COVID-19 is social and physical distancing. This means keeping space between you and other people outside your home.

This can be accomplished by working from home or staying home from work. It is seen with schools and universities, which are moving classes online, while doctors are treating via tele-medicine, and religious houses of worship are streaming their services online. Even restaurants are joining in the effort by offering take-out food or outdoor seating.

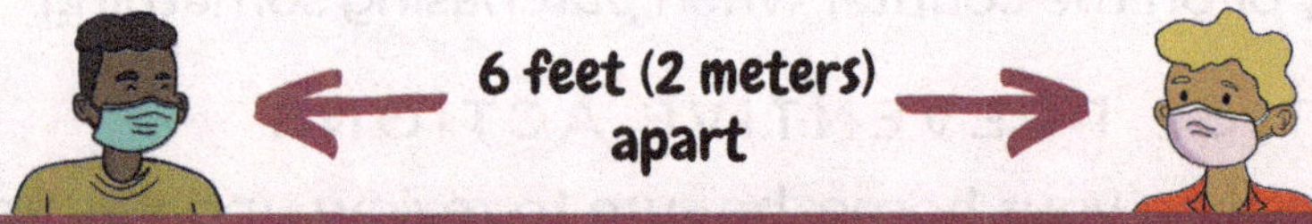

Important to note!

When dining out or eating with others, be sure to limit sharing items. Always inspect and ensure that what you are using is thoroughly cleaned and disinfected between uses.

We all need to do our part in stopping the spread of COVID-19 by practicing social distancing! This includes everyone; otherwise, it will not work. Keeping space between us and others is the best practice. We must avoid being exposed to the virus, while slowing its spread locally and across the world. There are indeed chances that you may have this disease for several days to weeks before showing any symptoms. Even if you are healthy, it is possible that you could transmit the disease while in close contact with others. While it may be hard to distance yourself from those you love, there are still ways you can be together.

Understanding the New Normal

COVID-19 spreads mainly when people are in close contact with one another for a period of time. Therefore, it is recommended to maintain at least 6 feet distance (2 meters) between you and the other person. You can measure the distance with an approximation of two arms' length.

Things you could do

Swap having coffee with friends for a virtual teatime hangout!

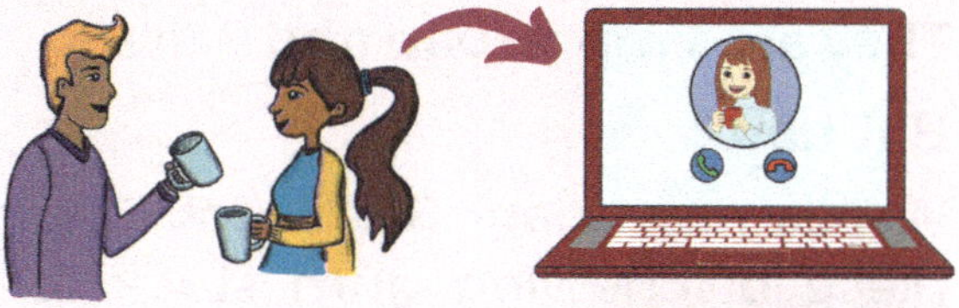

Swap a handshake for a hand wave!

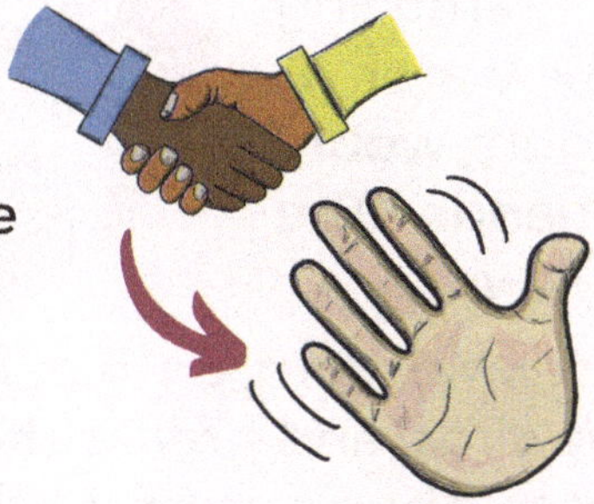

Swap face to face for facetime!

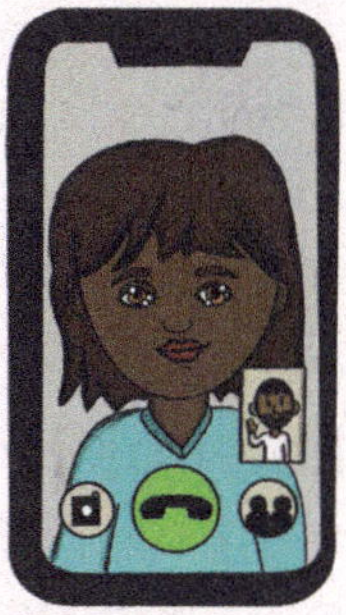

SAFELY LIFTING SOCIAL AND PHYSICAL DISTANCING RESTRICTIONS

As many states and countries ease restrictions and open economies, it is necessary to remain cautious. Opening up schools and businesses needs to be done gradually, or communities could face a tirade of new cases. Regulated precautions must be in place for all facilities, which include temperature checks, social and physical distancing, hand washing/sanitizing station, and access to masks if someone does not have one.

For normal activities to continue, it requires phases, discipline, and a gradual onset. Everyone has an important role to prevent the spread and protect themselves, their family, and the masses.

Hand washing and Hygiene

We all know by now that COVID-19 is a killer in some cases... but can we possibly kill it first?

The answer is yes! The weapons to kill COVID-19 are easily accessible, and can be found in our kitchens and bathrooms. They are simply soap and water!

But how?

We can compare SARS-CoV-2 with a piece of chewing gum stuck to our hands. Now, imagine removing chewing gum with simply water. It would flow over it, and the gum would remain attached to our hands. The same thing happens with the virus.

Virus

Like gum, a virus is actually very sticky, and likes to stick onto our cells

The virus is an invisible chewing gum on our hands. When using soap, it binds with the virus, and breaks the membrane open, killing it in the process. Then, water washes the virus into the drain, and bye-bye dead SARS-CoV-2.

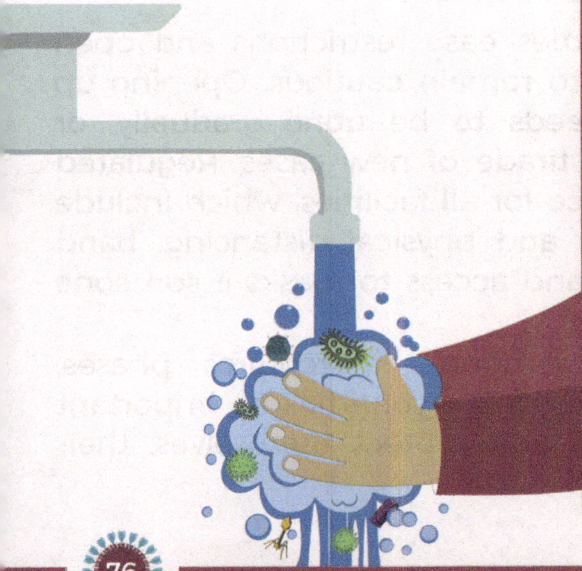

Always touching

Studies show that people touch their face at an average of 23 times an hour, including 10 touches of the nose, mouth or eyes.

SARS-CoV-2 spreads through these 3 main entry points, thus it is crucial to wash our hands with soap and water, which is the most effective way of preventing the spread of the virus.

HOW SOAP WORKS AGAINST COVID-19

SARS-CoV-2 molecule The virus uses its spike proteins to enter a cell and has a protective fatty acid membrane.

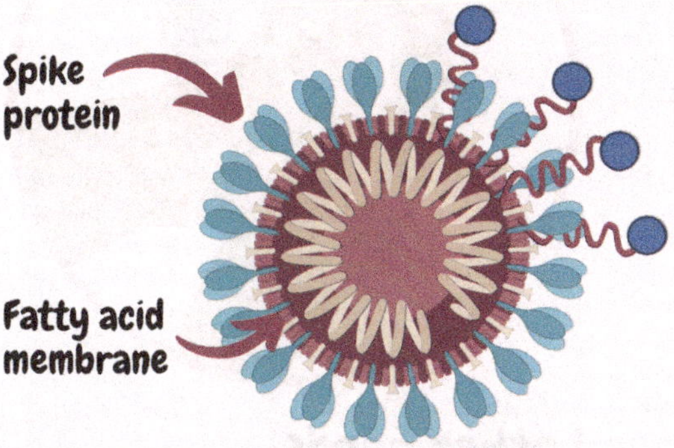

Soap molecule The head bonds to water and the tail avoids water

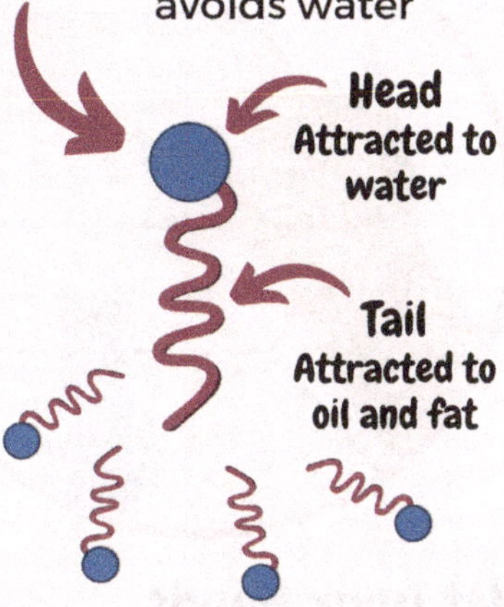

Soap molecule The tails of the soap (mixed in water) break apart the membrane.

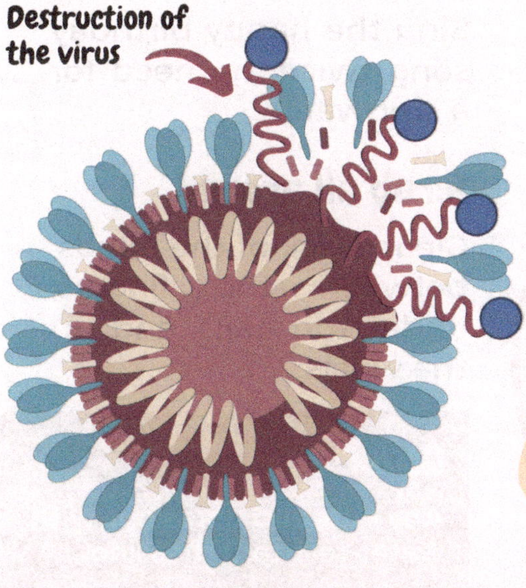

Bubble formation Soap surrounds the fragments of virus into bubbles called micelles.

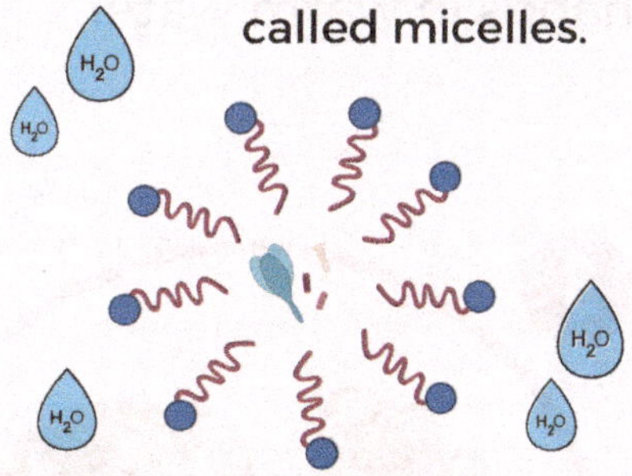

Bye Bye! The micelles are washed away by the water.

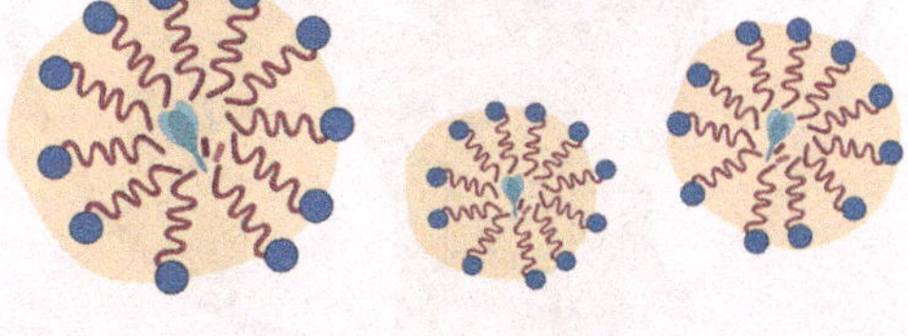

5 STEPS TO HAND WASHING

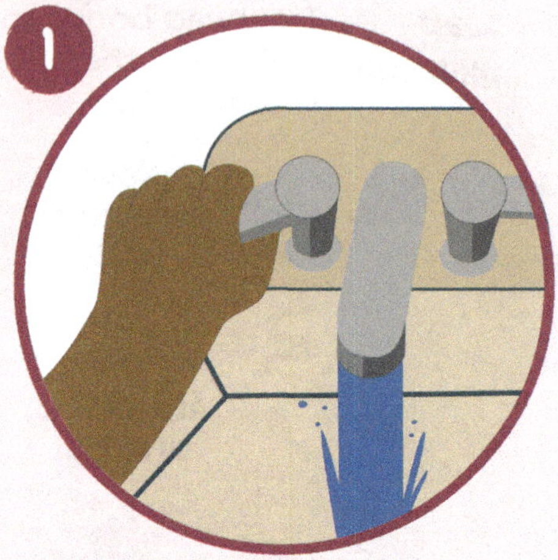

Wet your hands

Remove all jewelry and turn on the faucet to wet hands in warm water.

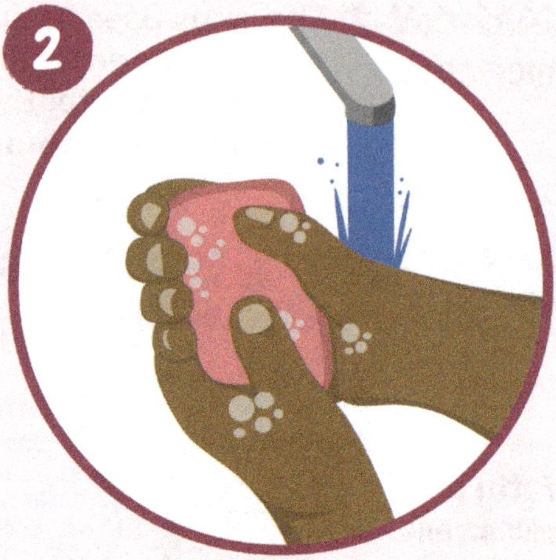

Lather hands

Use soap to create a thick lather for at least 20 seconds.

Sing the happy birthday song twice; no need for a stopwatch.

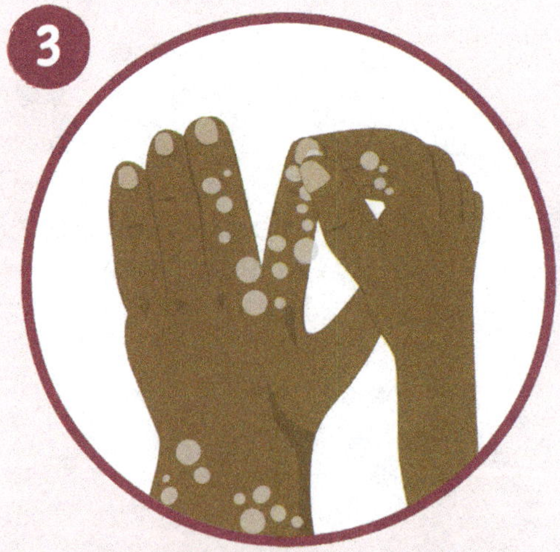

Scrub all around

Clean back of the hands, between the fingers, under the nails, and up the wrists.

Cover up

Any cuts and abrasions with water-resistant dressing.

Ouch!

Wash your hands as though you have just cut up chilies and wouldn't want them to go into your eyes.

4

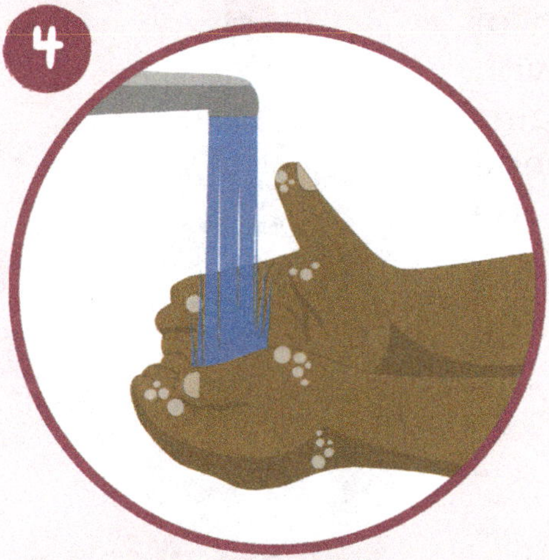

5

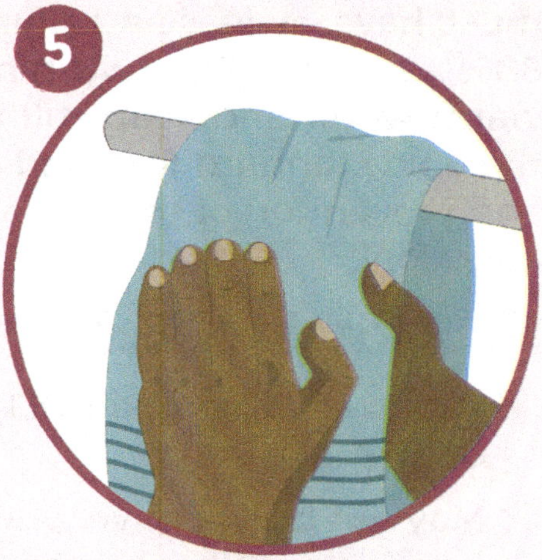

Rinse completely

Rinse off the soap thoroughly with clean and running water.

Beware!

DO NOT swallow, eat, or inject soap into your body in efforts to try to kill the virus. It does NOT work, and would instead send you to the hospital for serious complications!

Dry your hands

With a clean towel or air dryer.

Wash your hands

After you have been in a public place and touched a frequently touched surface, such as door handles, gas pumps, shopping carts, any electronic screens, etc.

Before touching any of the germ entry points: eyes, nose or mouth!

Alcohol hand sanitizer

When soap and water are not available, hand sanitizers are proven to be effective in reducing the number of microbes.

For the hand sanitizer to work, it must have at least a minimum of 60% alcohol. But washing with warm water and soap still remains the gold standard for hand hygiene and prevention of the spread of the infection!

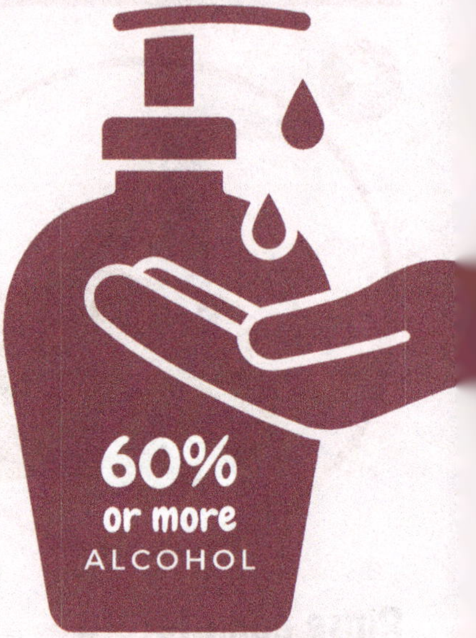

Not entirely effective

- Sanitizers **do not** kill all types of germs
- May **not** be effective when hands are visibly greasy or dirty
- Sanitizers **can** expire

Practice routine cleaning!

Clean and disinfect 'Frequently touched surfaces', such as, tables, light switches, remotes, door handles, desks, toilets, faucets, sinks, counter tops, and electronics.

Clean with detergent or soap and water before disinfecting.

Wear disposable gloves when cleaning and disinfecting; throw away gloves afterwards.

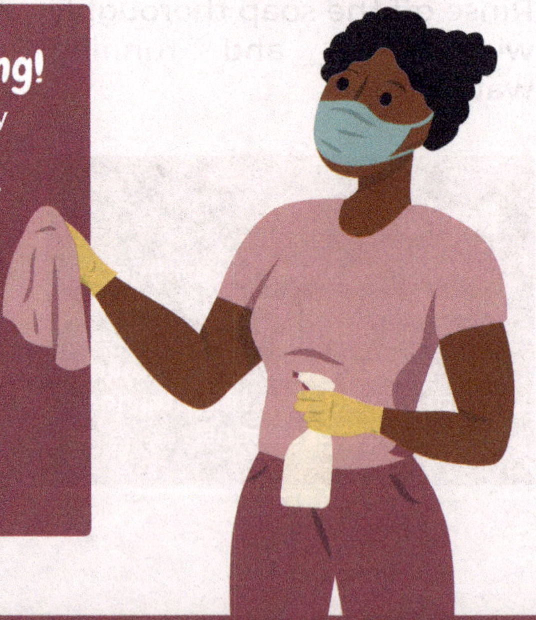

Reduce touching the T-Zone

Our eyes, nose, and mouth are our main entry points for COVID-19 into our body. We habitually touch this area without realizing it. For example, if we have an itch on our face, it's pretty hard not to touch and itch it. What we can do instead is try to itch it using the inside of our elbow, while keeping our hands away. We also have habitual actions, such as, nail biting, mustache twirling, or eyelid rubbing, which are hard to combat, but the best option is to create an alternative behavior.

Some options could be drumming our fingers on our thighs, or playing with a substitute object. Over time, these actions become habitual, and thus, we wouldn't need to worry about creating barriers to touch our face since it would just happen automatically.

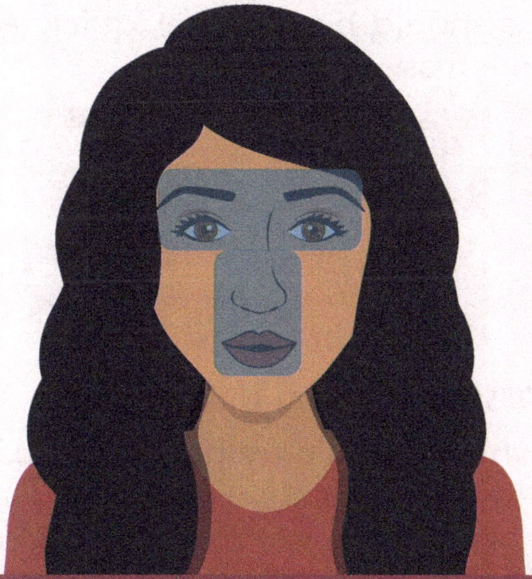

The T-Zone is the part of our face that makes up the forehead, eyes, nose, and area circling the mouth.

Quarantine

Quarantine is used to keep someone who might have been exposed to COVID-19 away from others. It is used to help prevent spread the disease that can occur before a person knows that they are sick, or if they are infected with the virus without feeling symptoms. While you are in quarantine, you should stay home, separate yourself from others, monitor closely your health, and follow directions from your state or local health authority.

Stay-at-home orders

Review updates from your local health authorities to understand what local orders are in place for your community. When staying at home, the best practice is to have a few weeks supply of medications, groceries, household items, and any emergency contacts. If you need to go out, the trips should be minimal, quick, and for essential purposes only, such as:

Food shopping	Medical assistance	Providing care	Donating blood
Volunteer and charity	Legal obligations	Access public service	Essential work

Seek medical assistance and isolate

Regardless of whether you have been diagnosed with COVID-19 or not, you should wear a mask when outside your home, and practice good hygiene outside and inside your home. If symptoms worsen, the best recommendation is to isolate immediately, and call your physician or seek a clinician via tele-medicine.

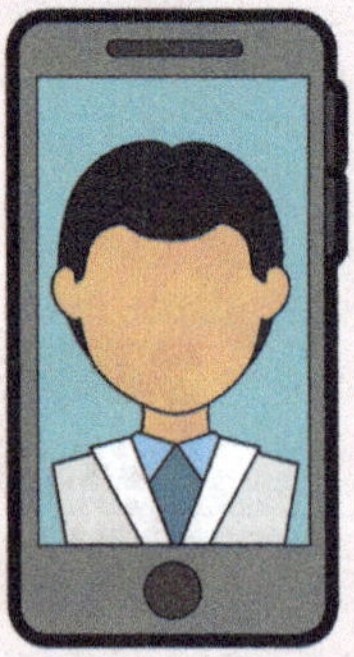

Isolation

Isolation is used to separate people infected with the virus (those who are sick with COVID-19 and those with no symptoms) from people who are not infected.

If you are affected and showing symptoms, it is best to isolate in a separate well-ventilated room, and if possible, use a separate bathroom. The key is to reduce shared activities with others; for instance, dining and close contact conversations. Be sure to also avoid sharing household items, such as, eating utensils, tooth brushes, towels, bedding, or clothing.

While in isolation, if possible, designate a healthy and chronic illness free family member at home to tend to your needs, such as, for food and essential items.

It can get lonely, but it is important to refuse all visitors!

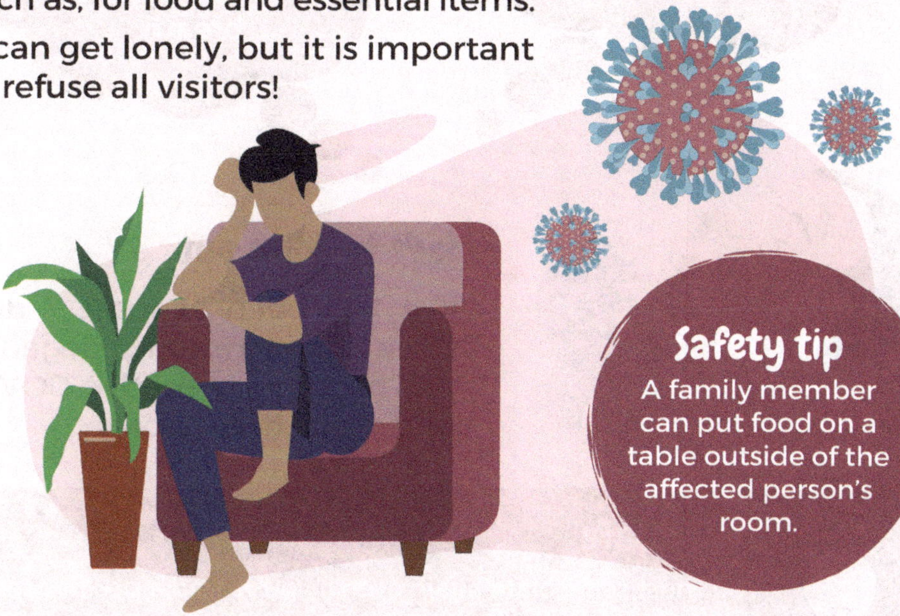

Safety tip

A family member can put food on a table outside of the affected person's room.

The caregiver should wear a mask when they are near you. And before and after any direct contact, the caregiver should wash their hands properly with soap and water.

How long should we isolate ourselves?

Speak to your doctor about how long you should isolate yourself.

Centers for Disease Control and Prevention (CDC) guidelines suggest the following to individuals coming out of isolation:

There is no fever for 72 hours (3 days) without using any fever reducing medication.

Symptoms are getting better such as cough and shortness of breath.

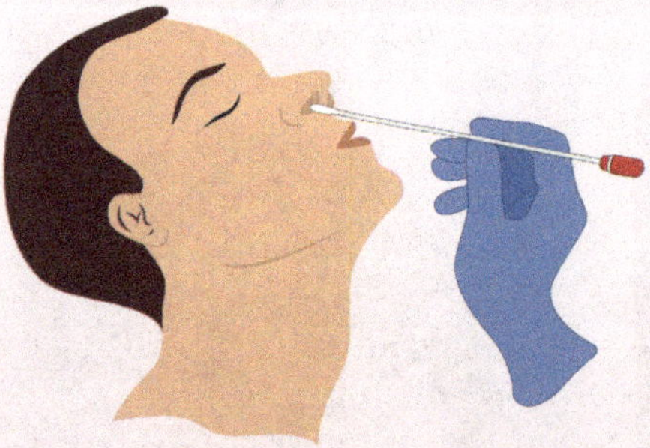

Safe to come out

If it has been at least 7 days since the symptoms began or you have two negative COVID-19 tests 24 hours apart.

Play it safe

You must self-isolate again even if you've had a positive test result for COVID-19 before. You probably have some immunity to the coronavirus but it's not clear how long it will last.

9 PPE: Personal Protective Equipment

- What is PPE?
- Types of PPE
- Masks

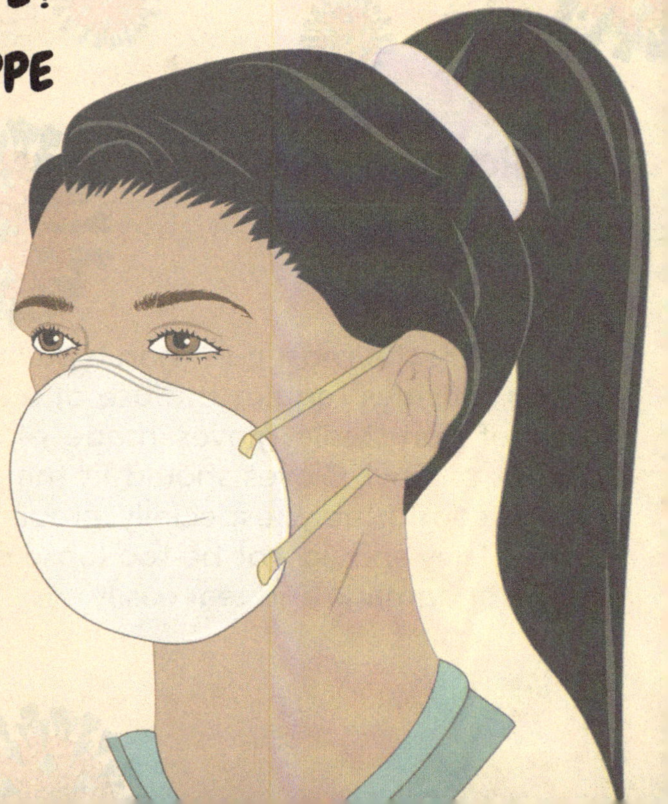

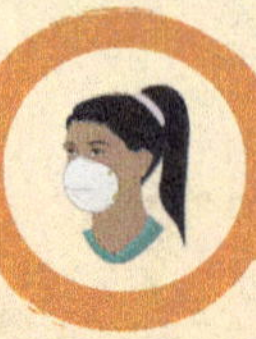

PPE: Personal Protective Equipment

What is PPE?

Personal Protective Equipment (PPE) is special equipment that is worn to create a barrier between us and the molecules that can possibly infect us. Especially in the hospital, the staff, including healthcare professionals, maintenance, and security, need their 'armor'. Just like soldiers at war, they are also on the frontlines during the pandemic. When selecting PPE, there are 3 key things to consider, namely:

- Type of anticipated exposure (e.g. touch, splash, large volume of blood/bodily fluid, etc.)
- Durability and appropriateness of PPE for the task (e.g. fluid resistant, fluid proof, etc.)
- Is it the right fit? (PPE size must fit the individual user)

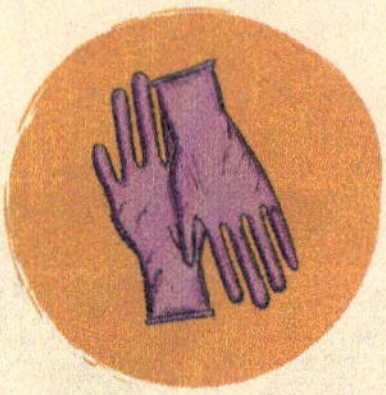

Gloves

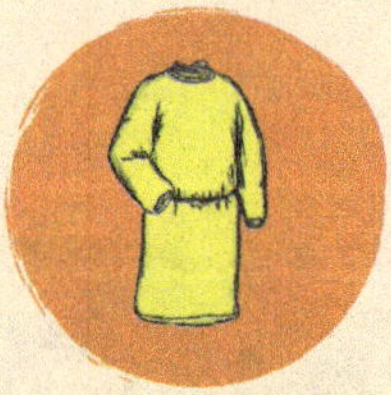

Clothing

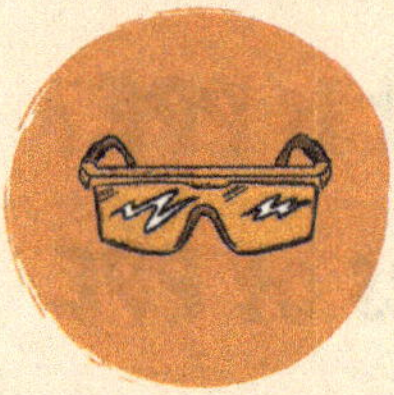

Eye safety

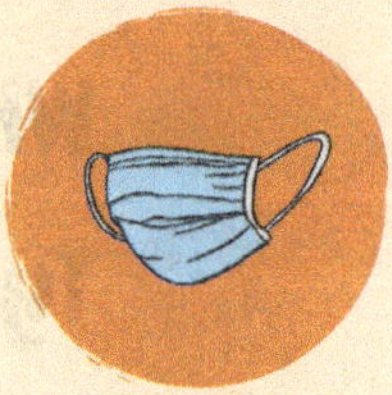

Masks

Types of PPE

GLOVES

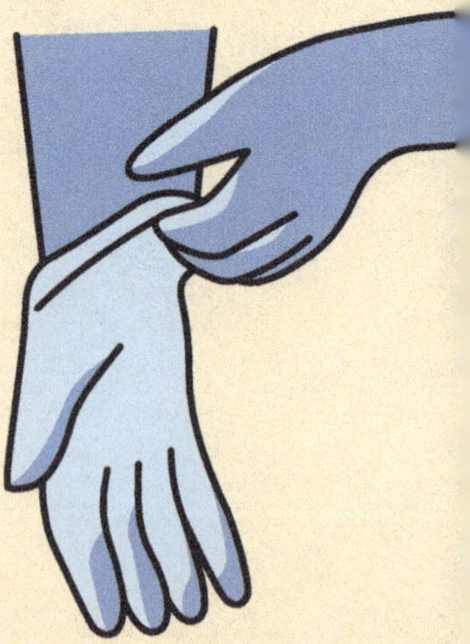

Gloves are the most common type of PPE. Most activities require the use of a single pair of non-sterile gloves made of latex, nitrile, or vinyl. Gloves should fit the user's hand comfortably, especially around the wrist. They should not be too loose or too tight, or damage and tear easily.

Especially in healthcare settings, gloves are worn for several hours, and thus need the reliability to take on the task. Gloves protect against contact with infectious materials. However, if contaminated, gloves can be the means of spreading infection to ourselves, other people, or on surfaces. Therefore, the proper use of gloves is crucial in order to be safe and keep others safe around us.

The Dos and Don'ts

The basic principle of infection control is to work from clean to dirty. This means touching the clean parts of the body or surface before touching the dirty or contaminated areas.

Therefore, limit opportunities for 'touch contamination', hence protecting yourself, others, and environmental surfaces. How many times do we see people adjusting their glasses, scratching their nose, or fixing their hair while wearing gloves? This is a form of touch contamination which can possibly expose you to infection. Always avoid touching unnecessarily anything when wearing contaminated gloves (e.g. light switches, cabinets, door knobs, etc.).

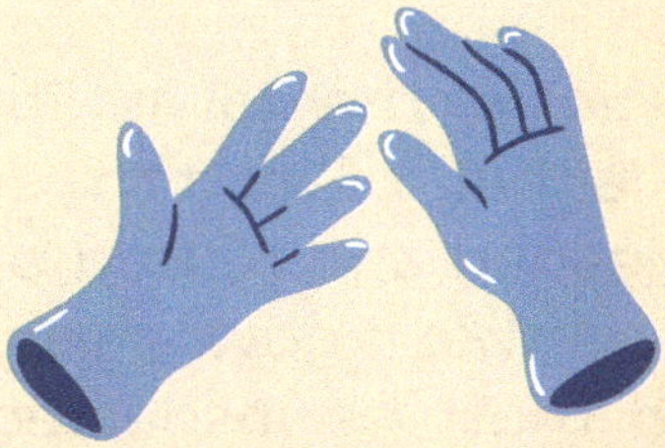

Always change gloves if torn or heavily soiled. It is important for healthcare individuals to follow this rule even if they are dealing with the same patient, and they should always change gloves when dealing with a new patient

Take note!

Gloves should never be washed and used again. Washing gloves does not make them safe for reuse. In fact, washing does not eliminate all the microorganisms, and makes gloves prone to tearing or leaking.

CLOTHING

Clothing consist of gowns, aprons, head covering, and shoe covers. There are gowns which are the preferred PPE, and there are aprons which are used when there is limited contamination.

Purpose of use

When selecting the correct PPE, if there is a risk for contamination of the arms, a gown should always be used.

Gowns should fully cover the torso

Have long sleeves covering the arms

Fit comfortably over the body and around the waist

Should have a snug fit at the wrist

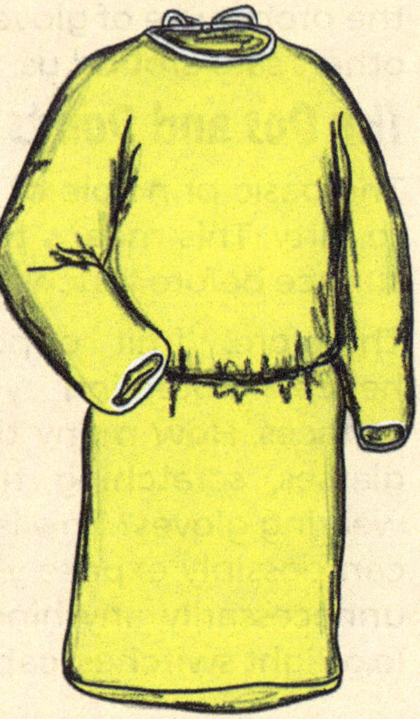

Material and Clean/Sterile

There are specific materials and properties of the gown. For example, isolation gowns are made either of cotton or synthetic material, and can be either cleaned and reused or must be disposed of. Cotton and spun synthetic gowns vary in their degree of fluid resistance, and must be inspected carefully when dealing with fluids that can penetrate.

There are two types of gowns – clean or sterile. Clean gowns are used for isolation, while sterile gowns are necessary when performing procedures or particular surgeries. The gowns ultimately serve specific purposes for the safe interaction between the patient and healthcare worker.

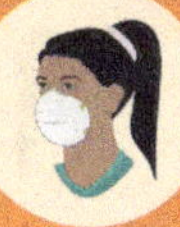

EYE SAFETY

A combination of PPE types should be available to protect all or parts of the face from any contact of infectious particles. Goggles or safety glasses are used to protect the eyes, and provide a barrier of protection of the mucous membranes through which germs can travel.

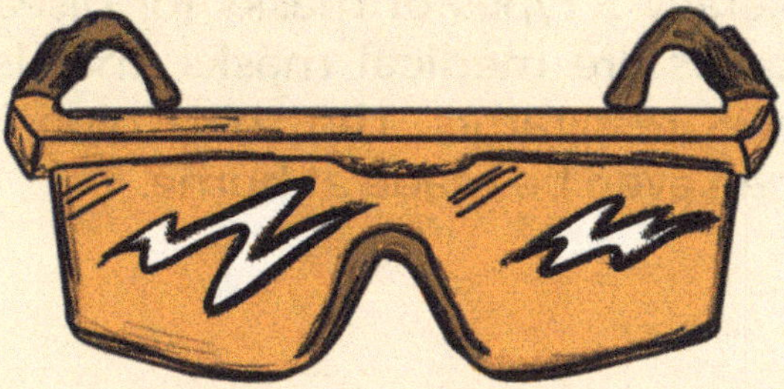

Should fit over and around the eyes

Personal glasses are not a substitute for safety glasses

Should fit comfortably over personal glasses

Face Protection

Face shields can be used in place or in addition to goggles and masks. They are used to protect the face, nose, mouth, and eyes. A proper face shield should cover the forehead, extend below the chin, and wrap around the side of the face.

Key points about PPE

- Wear it before coming in contact with the infected person
- When you have PPE on, use it carefully to prevent spreading contamination
- Remove PPE carefully and discard it
- Perform immediate hand hygiene

PPE: Personal Protective Equipment

Masks

When dealing with infections such as COVID-19, infection control reports state that droplets usually travel about 6 feet, which is about two arms' length distance. Masks are examples of PPE that are used to protect the wearer from airborne particles and from liquid contaminating the face. There are generally 3 types of masks for disease prevention. The 2 main types are medical masks, that is, surgical face masks, and N95 respirators. The third type is a cloth face mask, which can even be made at home.

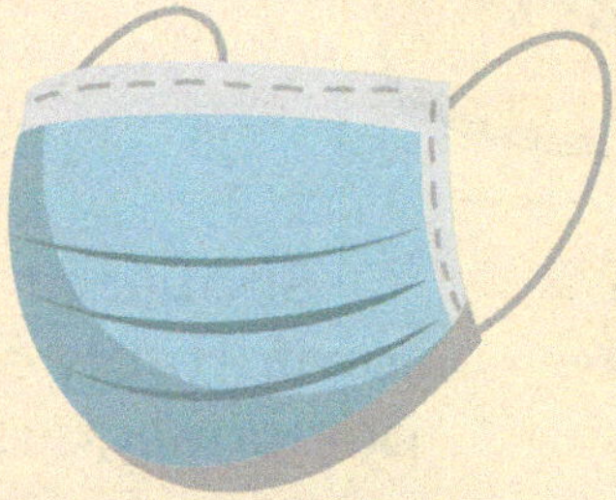

Surgical Mask

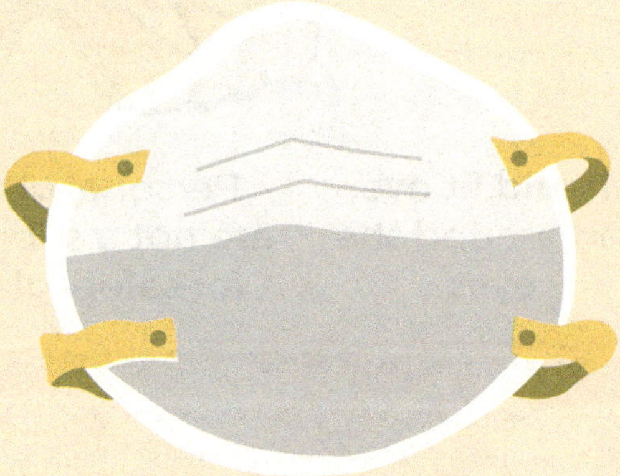

N95 Respirator

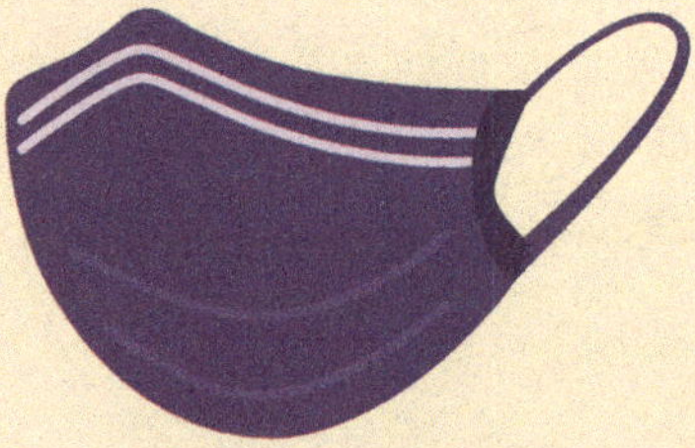

Cloth Mask

Use cloth face masks rather than surgical masks or N95 respirators as these critical supplies must be reserved for healthcare workers and other medical first responders.

All hospital staff, patients, and visitors should use PPE such as masks when there is contact with blood, bodily fluids, or risk of respiratory droplet infection.

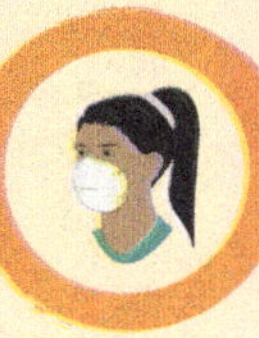

Cloth Masks

While surgical and N95 masks are in short supply, cloth masks are better than not using any mask at all. They offer some protection, are easy to find, and can be washed and reused.

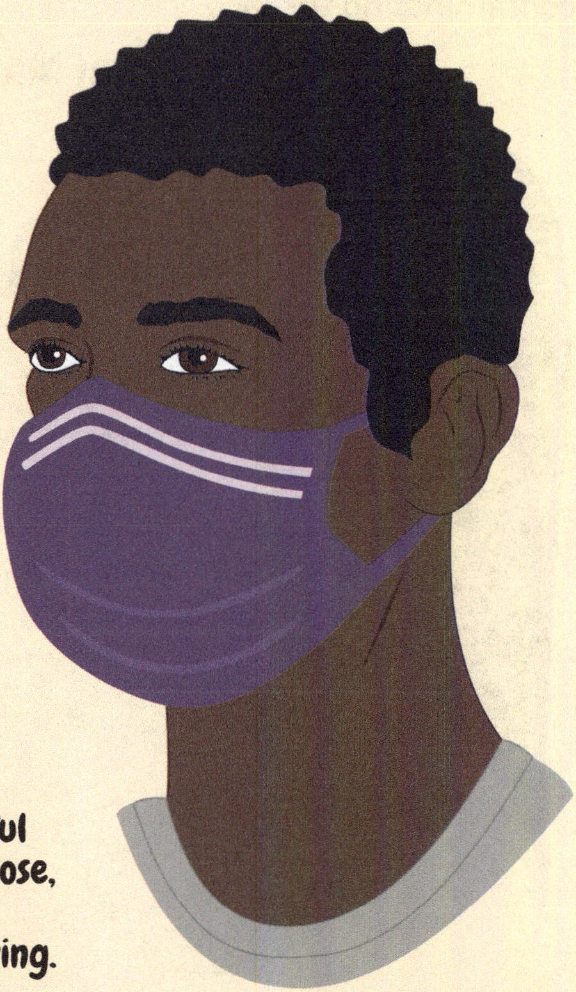

Wear in public settings, especially in populated areas

Don't put a mask on:

- Children under 2 years old
- People who have trouble breathing
- People who are unable to remove the mask on their own

Wash homemade cloth masks after every use

When removing, be careful not to touch your eyes, nose, and mouth. Wash hands immediately after removing.

They may provide a false sense of security. While homemade face masks offer some degree of protection, they offer a lot less protection than surgical masks or respirators.

Medical Masks

The 2 main types of medical masks are surgical face masks and N95 respirators. These are examples of PPE used to protect the wearer from airborne particles and from liquid contaminating the face.

Surgical Masks

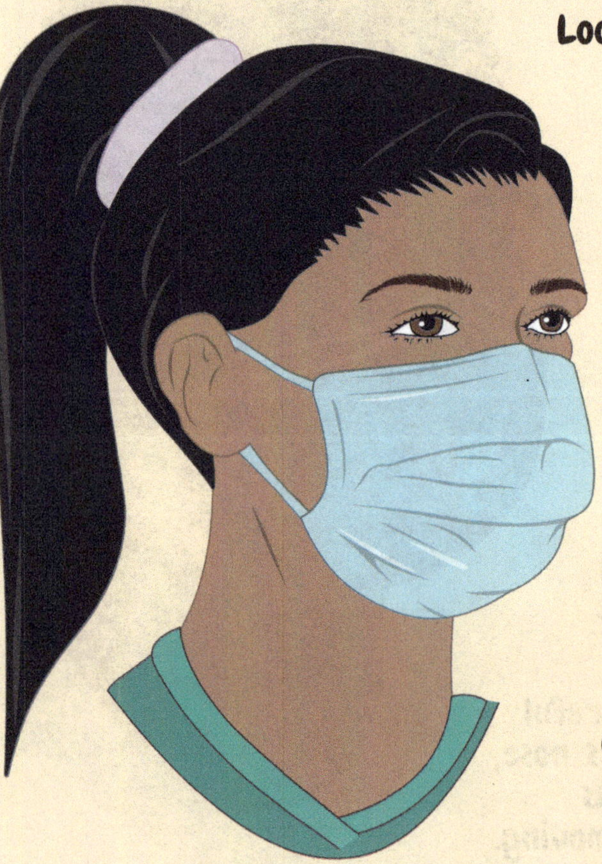

Looser fit and disposable

Create a physical barrier

Meant for blocking:

- Larger droplets
- Sprays
- Splashes
- Splatter

Prevent the wearer from spreading large sprays and droplets

May help reduce exposure of our saliva and respiratory secretions to others

They do NOT filter or block very small particles in the air when coughing or sneezing

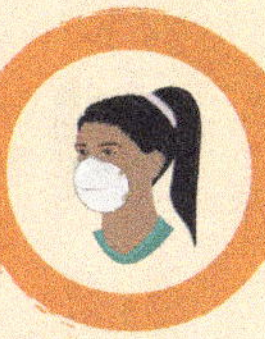

N95 Respirator

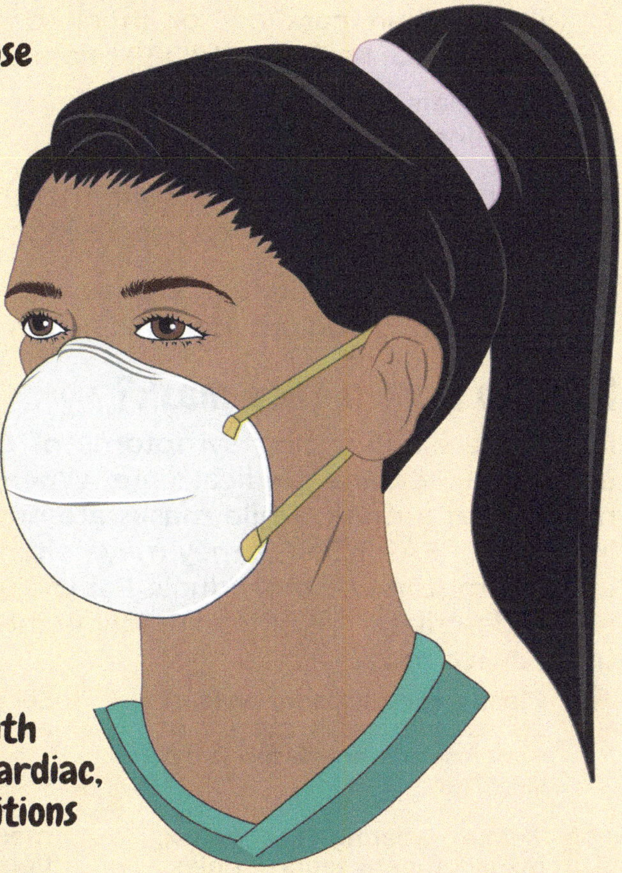

Tighter and a very close facial fit

Very efficient filtration for smaller airborne infectious particles

N95 means that the mask blocks at least 95% of small (0.3 micron) particles

Can make breathing difficult for people with chronic respiratory, cardiac, or other medical conditions

Please, first check with your healthcare provider

NOT recommended for general public use since it is required for healthcare workers and first responders!

Please note!
A properly fitted N95 respirator does not completely eliminate the risk of illness or death.

When to use a mask

- When taking care of or in close contact with a person suspected of having COVID-19 or another respiratory infection.
- Individuals with symptoms of respiratory infection, such as, coughing, sneezing, and/or fever.
- If you are a healthcare staff member, including security, maintenance, transporters and healthcare related positions.
- If the health authorities are recommend that it should be worn when going out in public places.

How do I use a face mask?

If you are experiencing symptoms of COVID-19, stay at home unless you require medical care. When going outside of your home wear a mask, while masks are not guaranteed to prevent infection of SARS-CoV-2, they may help prevent the transmission from asymptomatic individuals. For the optimal use of any of the masks described, it is critical to follow these general 8 steps when using a face mask:

1. Clean your hands for at least 20 seconds with soap and water or alcohol-based hand sanitizer.
2. Before wearing the mask, inspect for any tears or holes.
3. Orient the mask in the right direction. Locate metal clip for the top of the mask. For surgical masks - colored side faces outwards.
4. Place the top of the mask on the bridge of your nose, molding the fabric or metal strip to the shape of your nose.
5. Secure the elastic or straps around your ears or head.
6. Pull the bottom of the mask down to cover your nose, mouth and chin. Ensure a tight seal with no gaps.
7. Removing the mask: remove it from behind. Avoid touching the front of the mask, which may be contaminated.
8. Discard it immediately in a closed bin (or for cloth masks - put it in a sealed bag for washing) and thoroughly clean your hands for 20 seconds with soap and water.

10 Mental Health and Coping

- **Start your day off well**
  - **Mindfulness**
  - **Meditation**
- **Plan ahead**
  - **Do not overload information**
  - **Box Breathing**
- **Getting ready for bed**

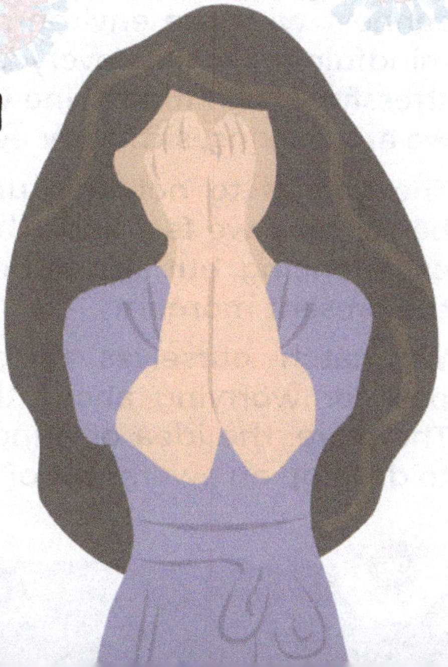

Mental Health and Coping

The COVID-19 outbreak can stir up all sorts of feelings, like fear, anxiety, or stress. A little stress can however be helpful. It can be the motivator that keeps us self-isolating or washing our hands. But constant or high levels of stress can affect negatively our mental and physical health. In the climate of a disease such as COVID-19, it harbors the power to destroy us mentally before it ever touches us physically. Therefore, the most important thing to do is 'protect our peace'.

Taking care of our minds and protecting our peace is always important, but doing so in the middle of a pandemic can be really tricky. Practicing certain techniques and applying recommended tips can help us all get through this.

Start your day off well

MINDFULNESS

It can be tempting to reach for our phone or switch on the news first thing in the morning, but starting the day with mindfulness can tap into our feelings, and allow us to connect with the environment around us. The practice of mindfulness makes everyday life more enjoyable and less stressful. It can intertwine with everything we do, whether we are walking, sitting, or even eating.

The goal is to not only understand better how we feel and what we are experiencing, but also to be aware of the present moment.

We catch ourselves replaying the past, or worrying about the future. Therefore, the idea of mindfulness is to develop an awareness of the now.

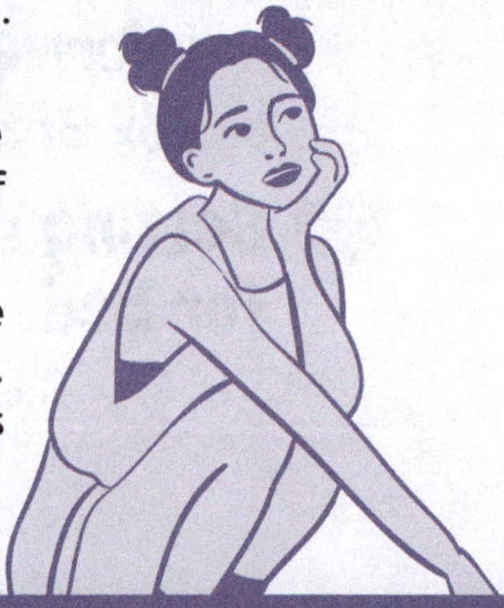

The 'Take in 3 things' technique can help us check in with how we are feeling and connect with our environment.

'Take in 3 things' takes less than a minute

LOOK

Before you get out of bed, pause, and concentrate on 3 things you can see. For example, look out the window at birds, look at your ceiling fan, or even simply look at your bed sheets.

LISTEN

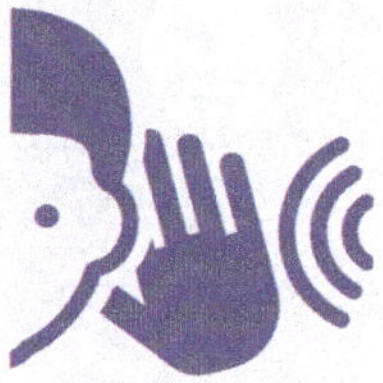

Now listen to 3 things you can hear. The birds chirping, sounds of cars passing by, or a lawn mower cutting grass. Capture it.

FEEL

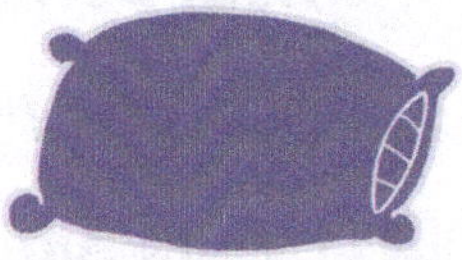

Finally, notice 3 things that you can feel in contact with your body. Your pajamas, the warm bed sheets, or the softness of your pillow.

There is no right or wrong in this technique; simply notice and be aware of what is going on around you, or happening in the moment. Let any or all things that you notice just be there. It sounds simple, but it takes effort, especially during difficult times like a pandemic when concerns about what the future holds generate unsettling feelings.

The technique helps train your mind to observe your own thoughts, feelings, and sensations with an objective view. It is easy to lose patience in the early stages of practicing mindfulness, so it is important to approach it with compassion.

MEDITATION

Believe it or not, our soul knows what to do to heal itself. The challenge is to silence the mind. With all the changes in our daily schedules and scare over the COVID-19 pandemic, stress and anxiety have a way of bringing us down. Incorporating meditation is a technique that takes just a few minutes, but has the ability to restore our inner peace, and provide tranquility in the long run.

Increase Gray Matter in Our Brain!

Recent studies from Harvard found that long-term meditators have increased amounts of gray matter in the insula, sensory regions, and the auditory and sensory cortex. Parts of our brain shrink as we grow older, which explains why we tend to forget things and slow down intellectually as we age.

Physical Benefits

- Boosts immune system
- Lowers high blood pressure
- Lowers the level of blood lactate, reducing anxiety
- Decreases tension-headaches, ulcers, insomnia, and other muscle pain
- Increases serotonin production - improved mood and behavior
- Efficiency of oxygen use in the body

Mental Benefits

- Stress & anxiety relief
- Increases creativity
- Develops intuition
- Peace of mind and mental clarity
- Increases focus which sharpens the mind
- Expands consciousness - leads to action/progress
- Reduces symptoms of panic disorder

"If you listen to your body when it whispers, you won't have to hear it scream."

MEDITATION IS BEING IN TUNE WITH OUR INNER UNIVERSE

Emotional

Stress reduction, lower blood pressure, immunity boost, pain relief, and heart health.

Unified Consciousness

We feel a connection with everyone and everything in our life.

Physical

Greater emotional balance, increased happiness, and a sense of well-being.

Witness Consciousness

We are detached observers, hence not as attached to things and outcomes.

Mental

Increased creative thinking, improved concentration, and increased productivity.

Wakefulness

We are more intimately present in the moment, and are more aware of ourselves and our environment.

How to do it

Daily practice of meditation improves your overall quality of life. All it takes is 5 minutes of your daily routine, and we have made it easy to practice in just 7 steps.

'Meditation in 7 steps'

1 SIT COMFORTABLY IN A QUIET SPOT

RELAX
Arms
Shoulders
Legs

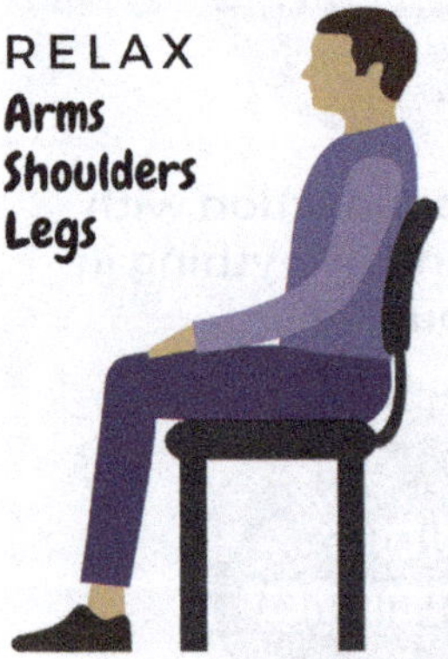

MAINTAIN
a straight & relaxed back

PICK
a good time and place where you won't be disturbed.

You can even try sitting cross legged on the floor!

2 FOCUS ON YOUR BREATH

FEEL
the breath going in and out.

PAY ATTENTION TO YOUR
Mouth
Chest
Abdomen

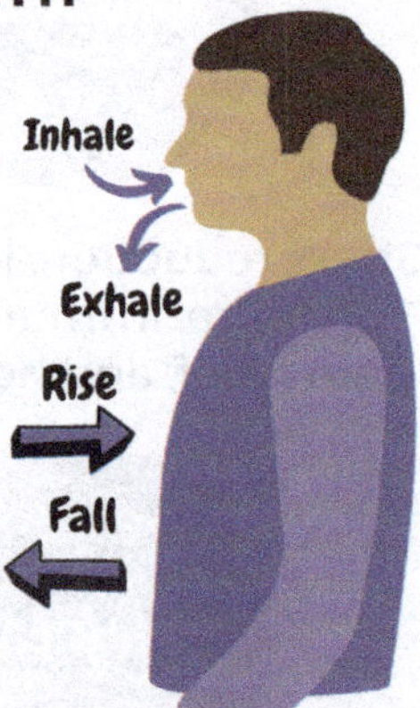

Count 1, 2, 3 during inhalation, and 1, 2, 3 during exhalation.

3 NOTICE EVERYTHING YOU'RE THINKING ABOUT

TRY LABELING
While simply observing your thoughts, it can be helpful to take it a step further and 'label it'. Say the words to yourself, or visualize it in writing.

DON'T FIGHT YOUR THOUGHTS

JUST OBSERVE THEM.

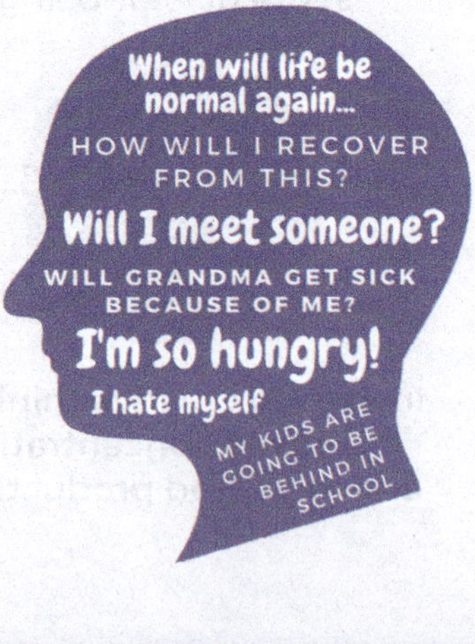

Your mind is full of thoughts, and it's NATURAL!

Mental Health and Coping

4 SLOWLY RETURN TO BREATHING

EMPTY
your thoughts, and live in the present by focusing on the breath.

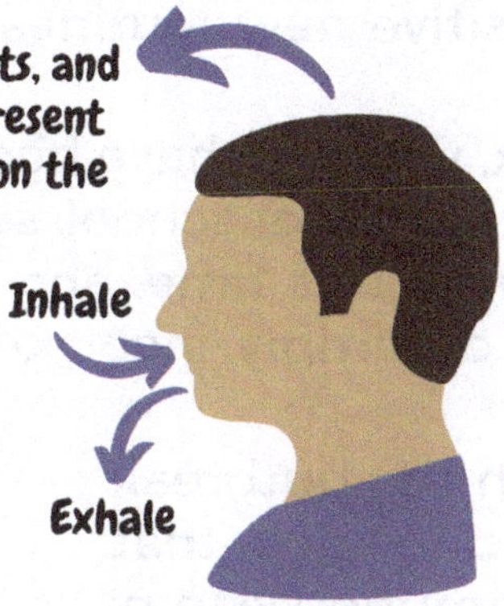

The empty mind is 'relaxed', it releases stress, and fosters well-being.

5 TRY TO DO IT FOR 5 MINUTES

OR YOU CAN
start with even less. Maybe try it for 1 minute in the morning.

WHEN YOU ARE CAPABLE OF
sitting still and relaxing for that long, move to 2 mins. Eventually, you'll get it.

If you have time to breathe, you have time to meditate.

6 NO DAYS OFF - PRACTICE EVERYDAY

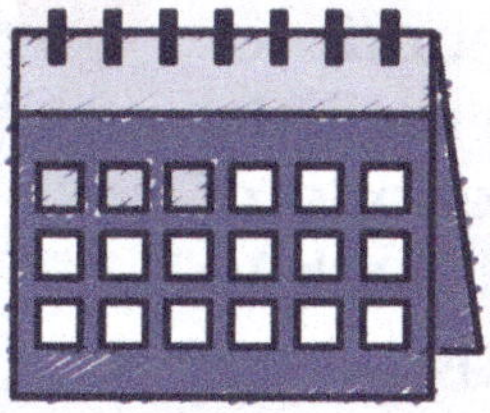

YOUR GOAL
is to make this a habit. The quality of the session will be better in due time.

TRUST THE PROCESS!

Frequency is even more important than duration.

7 PROGRESS TAKES TIME, SO BE PATIENT

YOUR AIM IS
NOT to control your thoughts, but to stop letting them control you.

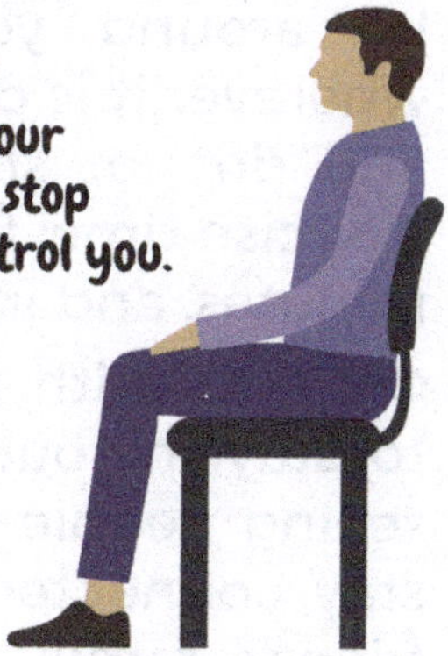

RELAX
in the present, unburdened by your thoughts.

Be here NOW. Be some place else later. Focus and meditate.

Plan ahead

We know how tempting it is to stay relaxed and lazy in bed, but adapting and creating positive new routines is helpful and keeps you motivated.

Prior to the COVID-19 outbreak, you may have been used to a 20-minute commute to get to work or school, such as, car ride, train, or even a walk. Mimic this time, and get some fresh air, listen to a podcast, or simply incorporate some sort of exercise.

Health anxiety has soared with the outbreak of COVID-19. However, it is good to know that exercising helps boost our immune system, improve mental well-being, and control weight gain. It is no surprise that obesity is one of the conditions that can worsen the effects of COVID-19.

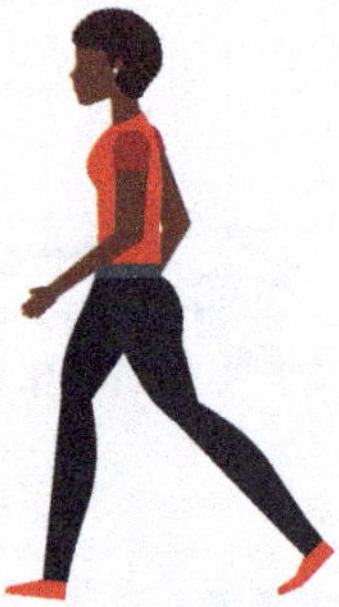

An easy way to start incorporating exercise is to simply walk. All you need to do is plug in a 10-minute walk into your daily routine. It can be around your yard, neighborhood, or wherever it is convenient for you. Be realistic, and do not shoot for extended periods of exercise time; first, challenge yourself with 10 minutes, and increase slowly as you go.

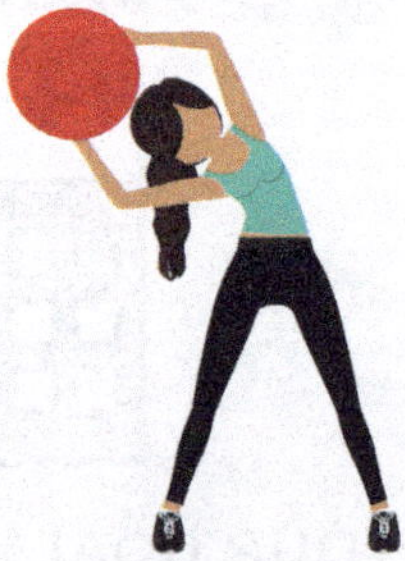

Connect with people. Sometimes, it is hard to stay in touch when we aren't physically seeing people every day. This is the time to stay connected. Set aside time to speak to friends, family, or work colleagues every day. The best way to release feel-good hormones is by connecting with people. These hormones are critical to relieve stress.

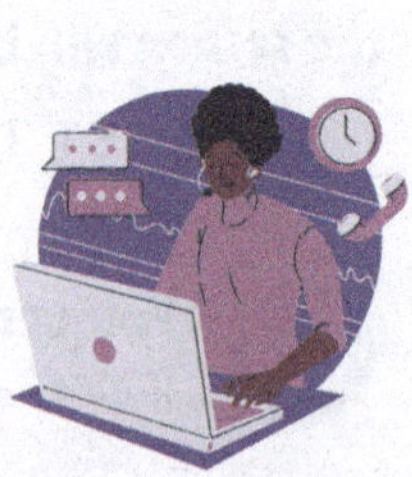

MAINTAIN SOCIAL CONNECTIONS

With the rise of COVID-19 cases across the world, it is understood there will be an increase in feelings of depression, anxiety, and stress. However, the concept of social isolation is often overlooked.

It is important not to confuse loneliness with social isolation. While they do intertwine, loneliness refers to the feeling of being alone, regardless of the amount of social contact. Social isolation is the lack of social connections. Social isolation can lead to loneliness in some, while others can feel lonely without being socially isolated.

Studies report that social isolation was associated with about a 50% increased risk of dementia, cognitive decline, cardiac issues, and a weakened immune system.

We as humans are generally social by nature, and maintaining social relationships can improve our overall quality of life, which even increases life expectancy. The practice of social and physical distancing does not have to result in social isolation. After all our biological systems and psyche has developed through social groups and the interaction between one another.

Social connections generate positive feedback loops of social-psycho and physical well-being. You can try:

- Connecting with friends, co-workers and family by phone or virtually through FaceTime, Zoom, WhatsApp, etc.
- Taking socially and physically distanced outdoor walks with friends.
- Making time for intimate conversations with people who you love and who care for you, such as family and friends.

DO NOT OVERLOAD INFORMATION

We are capable of coping with some stress here and there, but being overwhelmed with constant fear-inducing news feeds can be detrimental to our mental health. The stress response in our bodies happens when we hear upsetting or anxiety-provoking news.

Limit your news. Keeping informed is important, but managing your information intake makes a big difference in your overall state of mind. Limit reading or listening to news stories about COVID-19. Instead keep one or two reliable news sources, and check them once a day to keep informed.

BE OKAY WITH SETTING BOUNDARIES

Some people may ask you to hang out or go somewhere. During times like a viral pandemic, answering them is not an easy 'yes' nor is it an easy 'no.'

Cases in your community might be at a high or you might be living with someone who is sick or elderly. You may find yourself in a stressful situation in delivering a response to those extending the invitation. You may even ask yourself: Do I say 'yes' despite my concerns? Do I say 'no' without any explanation? Should I express COVID-19 related risks? Our response may come from societal pressure, social impression, or even obligation. But it is important to realize it is okay to set boundaries and be comfortable with an assertive response.

It's not an easy task but instead of feeling guilty or in distress when being assertive, try to accept the uncomfortable feeling. This will build confidence when giving responses.

Over time you will realize that saying directly what is on your mind, and what is important to you, will not only add value to your exchanges, but it will also make you feel good. Here are some examples:

"Thank you for the invitation, but I'm not comfortable attending at this time."

"You can visit, but I prefer to spend time in the backyard or outside."

"At this time I'm only comfortable with hanging out with family & a few specific friends."

"I'm okay with eating out at a restaurant, but we'll need to sit outside."

"I'm uncomfortable with having visitors, I'll let you know when I feel differently."

"I know the world has been scary, but I'll need to set limits on how much we talk about the news."

BOX BREATHING

If feelings of anxiety spring up in your day, try performing a breathing technique, such as, box breathing.
Box or square breathing is a technique used when taking slow and deep breaths. This technique is a strong stress reliever, and is beneficial to anyone wishing to reduce anxiety or worry.

It is also proven to be useful in heightening concentration and alertness.

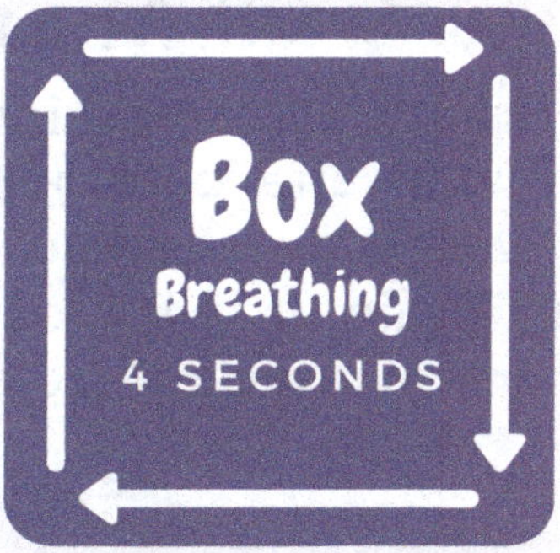

The best part is that it is quick, easy, and can be done anywhere.

How to do it

Before you start, make sure you are sitting straight up on a comfortable and steady chair. Place your feet flat on the floor and hands on your lap, with the palms facing up. Understand and feel your environment. Try to put all your focus on your breathing, and try not to have any environmental factors disrupting your focus.

Exhale Slowly

Empty the oxygen out of your lungs. Be conscious of your exhalation, and focus on the air coming out. You are now ready to begin.

Step 1: Nose Inhale – Take a deep breath in for 4 seconds

Using your nose - Slowly take a deep breath in for 4 seconds. Take your time when counting, and be conscious of the air traveling through your nose and filling your lungs.

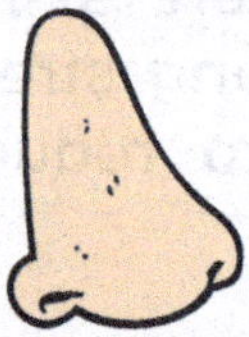

1 2 3 4

Step 2: Hold your breath for a slow 4 seconds

Holding our breath allows an increase in CO_2 retention in the blood, driving the cardio-inhibitory response of our vagus nerve when we exhale, and stimulating specific centers of our brain. It will create a state of physical and mental harmony in our body (relaxed & calm).

HOLD 1 2 3 4

Step 3: Mouth Exhale – Let the air out for 4 seconds

Using your mouth – Slowly let the air out for 4 seconds. Take your time when counting, and notice your abdomen and lungs working to push the air up and out of your mouth. Be conscious of your deep exhalation.

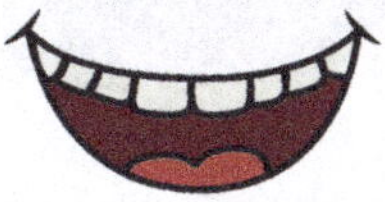

1 2 3 4

Step 4: Hold your breath again for a slow 4 seconds

HOLD 1 2 3 4

Benefits of Box Breathing

Box breathing is an effective and simple technique that restores your breathing to its best rhythm. Exercising it often is helpful for those who wish to reduce stress, improve future reactions to stress, and maintain overall positive mental well-being. It is recommended to individuals with depression, panic disorder, PTSD, or patients with advanced lung diseases, such as, Chronic Obstructive Pulmonary Disease (COPD).

- Calms the nervous system & relieves stress
- Increases mental clarity
- Reduces anxiety
- Enables better focus & retention
- Strengthens the ability to manage impulses
- Improves future reactions to stress indicators
- Relaxation response can reduce activation of genes associated with inflammation & stress

Getting ready for bed

Good sleep quality makes a huge difference in how we feel. Sleep can help our immune system function at its best. It helps us think clearly, be better at problem solving, and be able to deal with issues related to COVID-19. Additionally, adequate sleep aids in the stability of our mental health.

Feeling worried or anxious can make getting to sleep difficult. Lack of sleep is linked to depression, anxiety, and other mental health conditions.

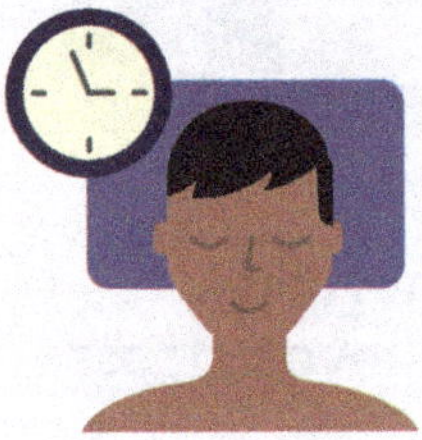

The best tip to getting good sleep is to follow a routine and stick to a schedule. One of the most important parts of your schedule by far is having a fixed daily wake-up time. Find a comfortable medium, and try to get at least 6-9 hours of sleep.

A bedtime routine should also be practiced. This involves a wind down time without any form of technology in the hours leading to bedtime. Avoid using your phone, tablet, computer or anything that has backlit. Its actually because our brain perceives the light coming from technology as day light and consequently suppresses the release of a hormone called melatonin, which helps put us to sleep.

Can't Sleep?

If you can't sleep because of constant stress and anxiety, try keeping a worry journal. This is where you can write down your concerns and all that is on your mind. Let go of those thoughts by writing them down, and then, put them away before bedtime.

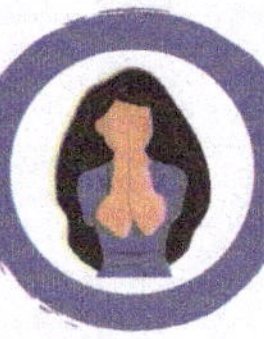

These practices help establish a connection with bed and sleep. The bed should only be for sleep and intimacy. If you are in bed, and you have trouble sleeping for 20 minutes, get out of bed and do something boring, such as, a puzzle, dim light reading, or an exercise. Once you become sleepy, you should now return to bed. You might also find it helpful to:

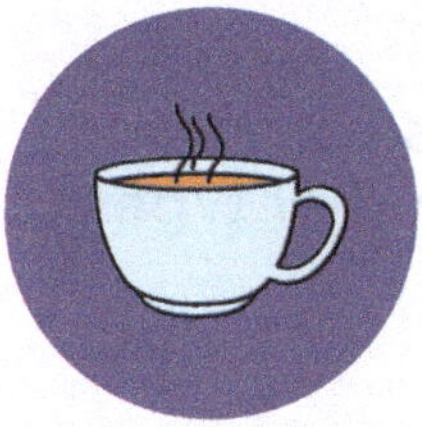

Avoid caffeine before bed

Limit food and drink intake late in the evening

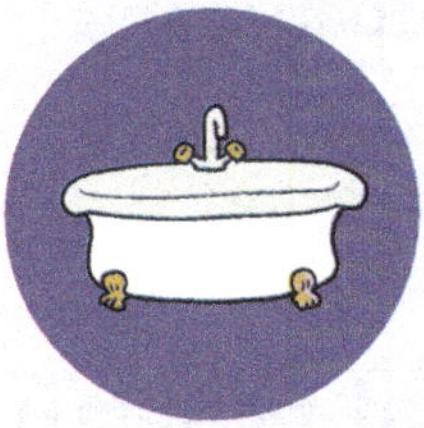

Take a warm bath

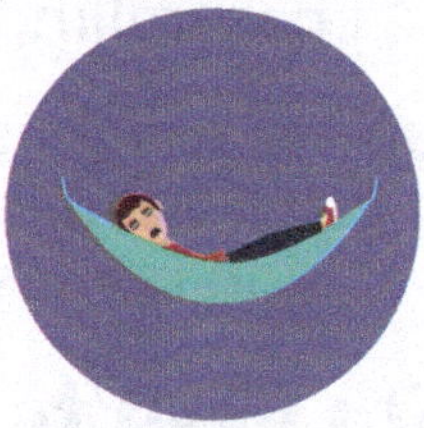

Avoid napping, or do it earlier in the day

Trouble sleeping? Try a 'Body Scan'

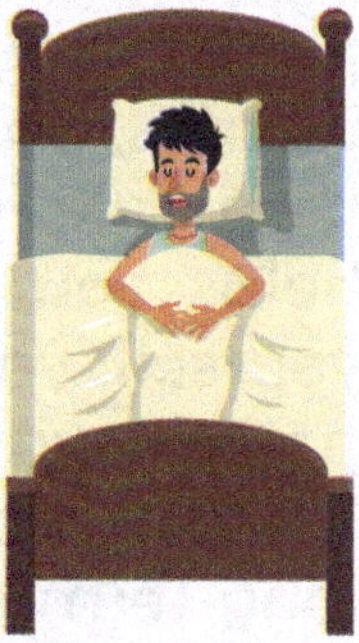

If falling asleep is becoming difficult, you can try doing a ‘Body Scan’. This simple technique can help you relax both your mind and body. With constant practice and consciousness, it can help send you off to a good night sleep.

How to do it

While lying in bed or resting, take your attention to your feet. Relax and soften them into the bed as much as possible. Then, scan up your body and move up to your ankles. Release any tension, and soften them into the bed. Once they feel relaxed, move up further to your calves, then knees, thighs, and so forth. Keep moving slowly up your body, all the way up to your head, softening and relaxing every muscle along the way.

Common signs of emotional distress

- Changes in appetite, energy, and activity levels.
- Difficulty and trouble going to sleep.
- Anger and issues with controlling situations.
- Headaches, body ache, stomach issues, and skin rashes.
- Inability to concentrate and pay attention.
- Avoiding activities that we typically enjoy.
- Returning to outgrown behaviors.
- Increased use of alcohol, tobacco, or other types of drugs.

It's okay to not be okay

It is natural to build up stress, sadness, anxiety, and constant worry during and after a major pandemic. All people handle these situations differently, and there is no perfect way of going about it. The key is to accept your worries, and take charge of self-care, or even seek out for help. Taking care of your mental health during a pandemic helps you maintain peace, and allows you to focus on yourself, your family, and loved ones. Most importantly, be patient with yourself. Self-care is tender; it is sacred ground. There is no greater investment, and it helps you in your long-term healing. Take charge of your mental health:

FIND THE RIGHT SPECIALIST

- ✓ Speak up if you need to see someone right away. Tele-counseling is widely available as well.
- ✓ Ask your primary health provider to help you find a specialist and make your first appointment.
- ✓ If the first mental health specialist is not a good fit, keep looking for one who works for you.

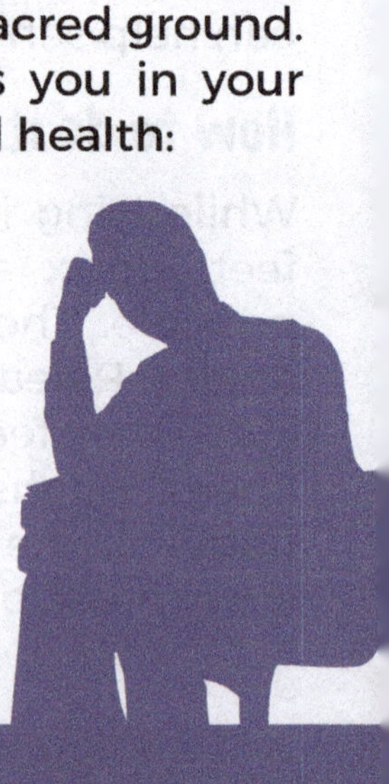

DEAR READERS

We would like to thank you for reading this book. When we sat down to write and illustrate the novel coronavirus, we kept in mind how this guide can benefit you. With so many amazing resources and content displayed by writers and creators across the world, we wanted to make sure that we added value to your decision to spend time reading this book.

Thank you for appreciating why this guide matters. You matter, and your effort to understand COVID-19 really matters. In many ways, writing a book about a disease affecting us all is much like teamwork, and in order for the world to heal, we must all work together to help one another. We are alone together.

We thank you for sharing this book with colleagues, friends, and family. It took time and effort to showcase the pandemic and all the necessary information in each chapter. However, through this journey, there was something beautiful that we saw...so many talented individuals from different nations across the world offered their expertise, time, and effort to ensure that this guide became a reality. And this restores our hope in humanity.

There is still much more to understand about the virus that caused the earth to stand still. We promise to continue writing, and join our courageous frontline healthcare workers in the pursuit of a safer, healthier, and better tomorrow.

Thank you, readers. We really thank you,

Syed, Pippa, Rebecca, Daniel

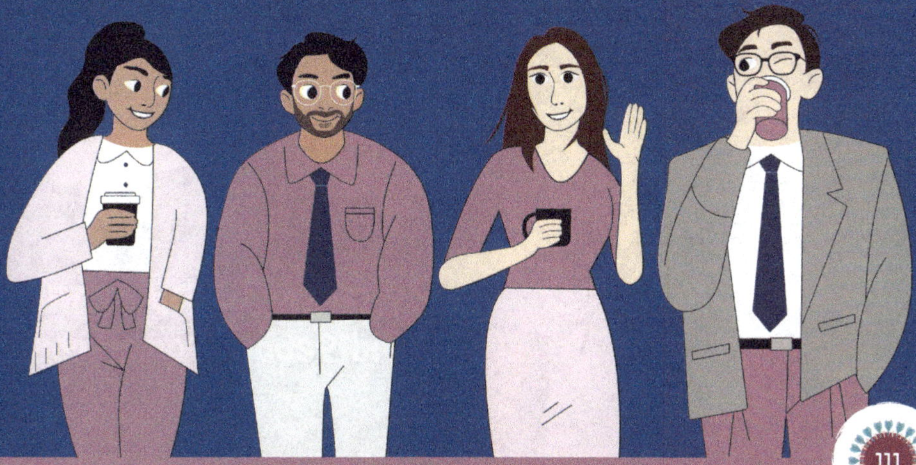

WEBSITE

FOR MORE INFORMATION ABOUT THE BOOK, PLEASE VISIT:

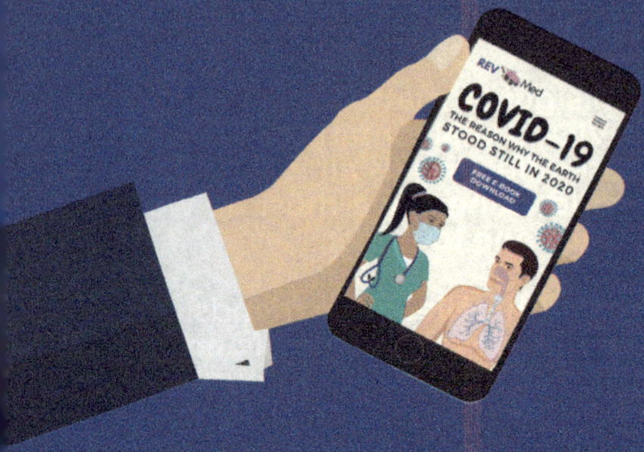

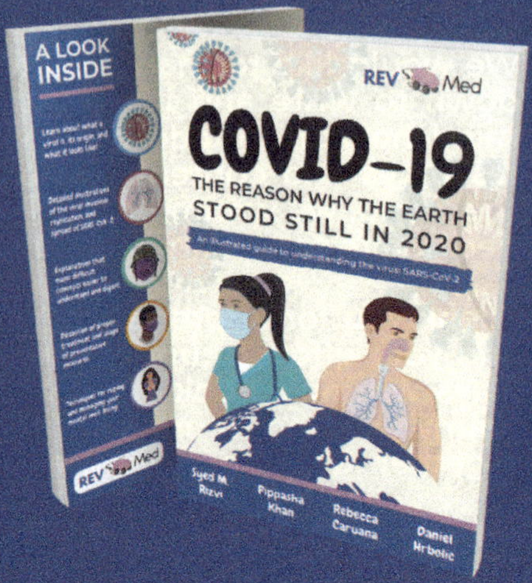

www.covid19ebook.org

CONTACT US

Send us a message.

The good ones will go viral.

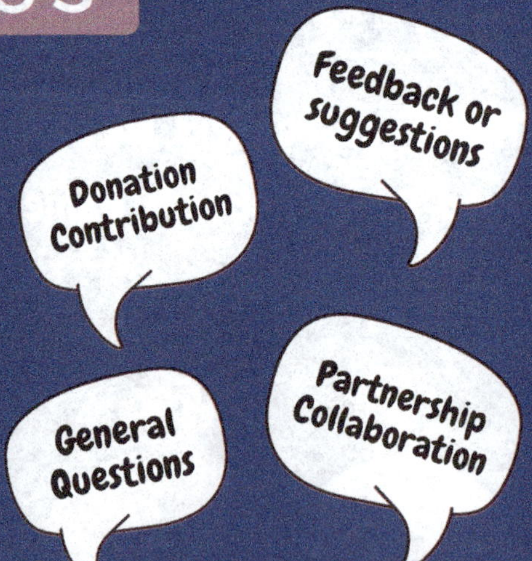

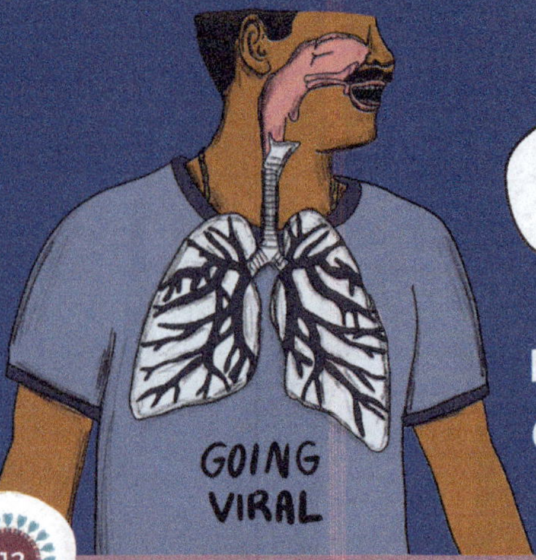

Message us by email

covid19ebook@gmail.com

HELP US WRITE MORE BOOKS

Make a One-Time Donation

We have proudly written this book for anyone around the world to access it. This was possible by making sure it is **100% FREE** of cost to download. We did this because we understand during difficult times, comes financial burden, and many across the world do not have the means to afford literature. We, the authors, firmly believe in the access to healthcare literature for all.

In the near future, we hope to release health-related books for healthcare students, the general public, and even children! Undoubtedly, our pride will always be in maintaining the highest quality of work.

You can help write these books by donating today!

We are collecting funds to:

- Print hard copies of this book
- Have the book translated into multiple languages
- Donate print copies to lower socio-economic areas
- Prospect only the best illustrators, designers, and medical professionals to write

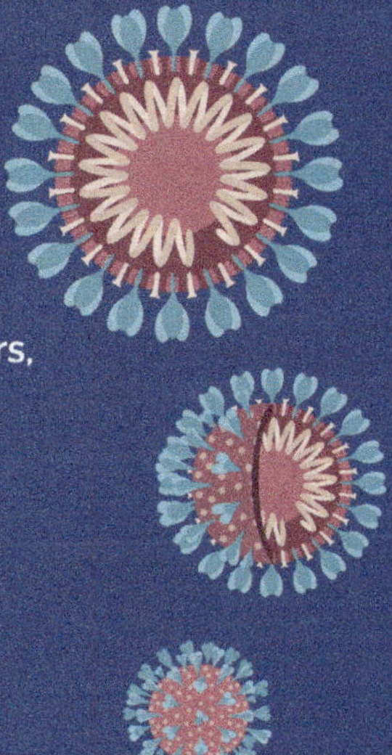

Donate now

Visit: www.covid19ebook.org

Whether you are able to give enough for a coffee or completely fund the next book, we promise that each and every donation goes a long way. We will rely on each other to carry out the mission to produce health literature, and keep it accessible and free.

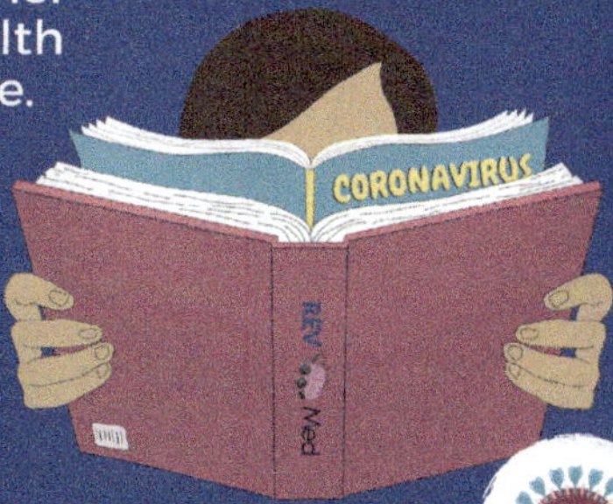

For questions regarding donations and contributions, please feel free to contact us!

covid19ebook@gmail.com

REFERENCES

Note: Information found throughout this guide book is sourced and reported from credible institutions, organizations and, health authorities. You can find more information by clicking any of the links below.

Disclaimer: This guide book is for informational purposes only, it is not to substitute a health expert's or medical professional's advice.

WHO: World Health Organization

CDC: Centers for Disease Control and Prevention

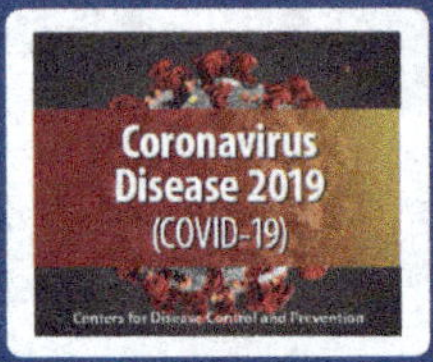

NIH: National Institutes of Health | Coronavirus (COVID-19)

FDA: U.S. Food & Drug Administration | Coronavirus Disease 2019 (COVID-19)

UN: United Nations | COVID-19 Response

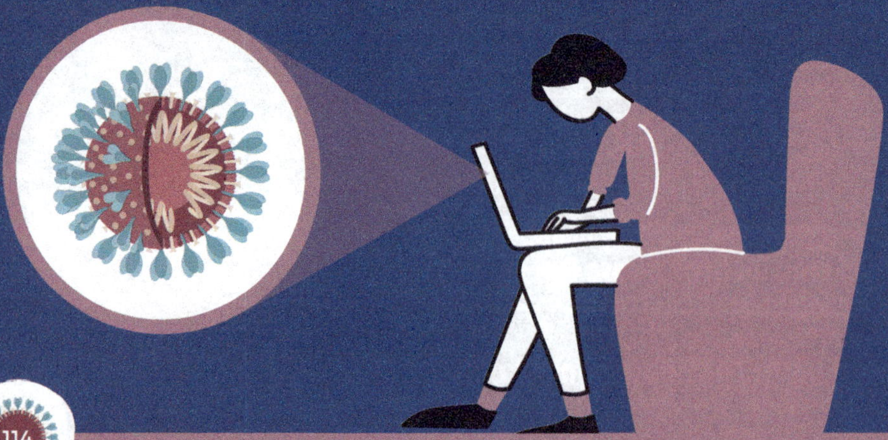

TEAM AND COLLABORATION

Meaden Creative

GRAPHIC DESIGN

www.meadencreative.com

LONDON, UK

Lilly Air

ILLUSTRATOR
FRONTISPIECE DESIGN

@lillyair

ACADEMY OF ART UNIVERSITY
SAN FRANCISCO, CA, US

WWW.LILLYAIR.COM

Constantine Suvorov

TV NETWORK ENGINEER
APP DEVELOPMENT

REV MED | MEDICINE ALIVE

KSUVORAU@GMAIL.COM

Zulfiqar Rizvi

CONTENT DEVELOPER
MARKETING & DESIGN

@zfilms

ZFILMS
NEW YORK, NY, US

Ingenious Guru

WEBSITE DESIGN & MANAGEMENT
DIGITAL MARKETING AGENCY

@Ingeniousguru

INGENIOUS GURU
OHIO, US

WWW.INGENIOUSGURU.COM

Christina Santos

GRAPHIC DESIGNER
LAYOUT DESIGN

@headinacanvas

FASHION INSTITUTE OF TECHNOLOGY
NEW YORK, NY, US

Medical Mnemonics

MEDICAL EDUCATION ON SOCIAL MEDIA

@mnemonicsmed

USEFUL RESOURCES

CDC: Centers for Disease Control and Prevention

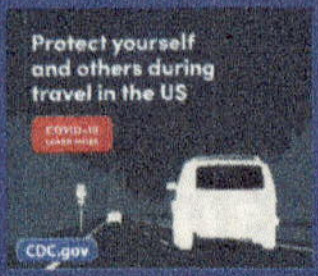

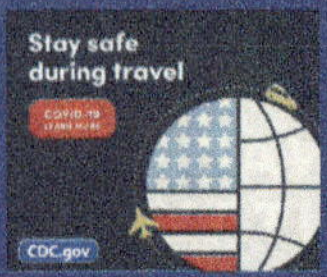

NIH: National Institute on Drug Abuse

Individuals dealing with substance use disorders and in recovery.

NAMI: National Alliance on Mental Illness

COVID-19 Resource and Information Guide

WHO: World Health Organization

COVID-19: Resources for Pregnancy, Childbirth, Postnatal Care

FDA: U.S. Food & Drug Administration

Multilingual COVID-19 Resources

NASN: National Association of School Nurses

Resources and Guidance for returning to school

The White House

Coronavirus (COVID-19)

FREE U.S. COUNSELING

National Suicide and Crisis

National Suicide Prevention Lifeline

(800) 273-8255

Free and confidential 24/7 support, information and resources.

Ayuda En Espanol

(888) 628-9454

Llama a este número para ayuda 24/7 en español del National Suicide Prevention Lifeline.

Crisis Call Center

(800) 273-8255

Safe source of support for individuals in any type of crisis. 24/7/365 support.

YouthLine

(877) 968-8491

Call or text teen2teen to 839863 to recieve teen-to-teen crisis support during select hours and adult support at all other hours.

USEFUL RESOURCES

Domestic and Sexual Violence

National Domestic Violence Hotline

(800) 799-7233

If you're unable to speak safely, you can log onto thehotline.org or text LOVEIS to 22522

The National Sexual Assault Telephone Hotline

(800) 656-HOPE (4673)

Be connected with a trained staff member from a sexual assault service provider in your area.

Take the Night Foundation Hotline

(547) 742-8837

24/7 hotline for free legal advice, support, and information from volunteer attorneys who specialize in free legal assistance for sexual and domestic abuse survivors

Elder Abuse Hotlines

(800) 677-1116

If you suspect elder abuse, neglect, or exploitation, call your state's elder abuse hotline by calling the number above.

Alcohol and Substance Abuse

SAMHSA's National Helpline

(800) 662-4357

Free, confidential, 24/7/365 mental health and substance use disorder treatment, referral, and information service. (Eng and Spanish)

Narcotics Anonymous

(818) 773-9999

Call the NA World Services line for general information about Narcotics Anonymous and its mission to support people seeking recovery from addiction.

Alcoholics Anonymous

(212) 870-3400

Call the AA World Services line for general information about Alcoholics Anonymous and its mission to support people seeking recovery from alcohol addiction.

The Partnership for Drug-free Kids Helpline

(855) 378-4373

If you are having difficulty accessing support for your family, or a loved one struggling with addiction or treatment challenges resulting from COVID-19 circumstances, specialists here can guide you.

Mental Health and Support

SAMHSA's National Helpline

(800) 662-4357

Free, confidential, 24/7/365 mental health and substance use disorder treatment referral and information service. (Eng and Spanish)

NeedyMeds

(800) 503-6897

Call for information about patient assistance programs and other ways to get help covering the cost of medication.

USEFUL RESOURCES

National Institute of Mental Health Information Center

(866) 615-6464

Call for information about mental health conditions and updates on the latest advancements in mental health treatment and research.

NAMI: National Alliance on Mental Illness Helpline

(800) 950-6264

If you or a loved one are living with a mental illness and need help, call the NAMI Helpline for information, resource referrals, and support.

Grief Support

GRASP: Grief Recovery After a Substance Passing

(302) 492-7717

Call to learn more about their mission to support people who have lost someone to substance use or addiction. Find local meetings.

GriefShare

(800) 395-5755

Contact to learn more about their mission to connect people who are grieving with one another.

MADD: Mothers Against Drunk Driving

(877) 623-3435

Call the MADD 24-hour Victim Help Line for support if you have lost a loved one to a drunk driving accident.

Caregiver Help Desk

(855) 227-3640

Navigate your complex caregiving challenges with experts. Find tips for family caregivers and COVID-19.

Organizations

Centers for Disease Control and Prevention

(800) 232-4636

As the US health protection agency, CDC saves lives and protects people from health, safety, and security threats.

World Health Organization

1211 Geneva
+41-22-7912111

WHO works worldwide to promote health, keep the world safe, and serve the vulnerable.

Pan American Health Organization

(202) 974-3000

PAHO is the specialized international health agency for the Americas. It works with countries throughout the region to improve and protect people's health.

National Health Service

0300 311 22 33

NHS' aim is to deliver the right care to the right people at the right time. Our mission is to improve health and secure high quality healthcare for the people of England, now and for future generations

CHECKLIST FOR BACK TO SCHOOL

*PARENTS CAN USE THIS CHECKLIST FOR CHILDREN RETURNING BACK TO CLASSES. CDC.GOV/CORONAVIRUS

Actions to take and points to consider	Notes
☐ Check in with your child each morning for signs of illness. If your child has a temperature of 100.4 degrees or higher, they should not go to school. ☐ Make sure your child does not have a sore throat or other signs of illness, like a cough, diarrhea, severe headache, vomiting, or body aches. ☐ If your child has had close contact to a COVID-19 case, they should not go to school. Follow guidance on what to do when someone has known exposure.	
☐ **Identify** your school point person(s) to contact if your child gets sick.	Name of school point person(s): Contact info:
☐ **Make sure** your child is up-to-date with all recommended vaccines, including for flu. All school-aged children should get an influenza flu vaccine every season, with rare exceptions. This is especially important this year because we do not yet know if being sick with COVID-19 at the same time as the flu will result in more severe illness.	Date of flu vaccination:
☐ **Be familiar** with local COVID-19 testing sites in the event you or your child develops symptoms.	My local testing options:

CHECKLIST FOR BACK TO SCHOOL

*PARENTS CAN USE THIS CHECKLIST FOR CHILDREN RETURNING BACK TO CLASSES. CDC.GOV/CORONAVIRUS

Actions to take and points to consider	Notes
☐ **Review and practice** proper hand washing techniques at home, especially before and after eating, sneezing, coughing, and adjusting a mask. Make hand washing fun and explain to your child why it's important.	
☐ **Be familiar** with how your school will make water available during the day. Consider packing a water bottle.	
☐ **Develop** daily routines before and after school—for example, things to pack for school in the morning (like hand sanitizer and an additional (back up) mask) and things to do when you return home (like washing hands immediately and washing masks).	
☐ **Talk** to your child about precautions to take at school. Children may be advised to: • Wash and sanitize their hands more often. • Keep physical distance from other students. • Wear a mask. • Avoid sharing objects with other students, including water bottles, devices, writing instruments, and books. • Use hand sanitizer (that contains at least 60% alcohol.) Make sure you're using a safe product. FDA recalled products that contain toxic methanol. Monitor how they feel and tell an adult if they are not feeling well.	

CHECKLIST FOR BACK TO SCHOOL

*PARENTS CAN USE THIS CHECKLIST FOR CHILDREN RETURNING BACK TO CLASSES. CDC.GOV/CORONAVIRUS

Actions to take and points to consider	Notes
☐ **Develop** a plan as a family to protect household members who are at increased risk for severe illness.	
☐ **Make sure** your information is current at school, including emergency contacts and individuals authorized to pick up your child(ren) from school. If that list includes anyone who is at increased risk for severe illness from COVID-19, consider identifying an alternate person.	
☐ **Be familiar** with your school's plan for how they will communicate with families when a positive case or exposure to someone with COVID-19 is identified and ensure student privacy is upheld.	
☐ **Plan** for possible school closures or periods of quarantine. If transmission is increasing in your community or if multiple children or staff test positive for COVID-19, the school building might close. Similarly, if a close contact of your child (within or outside of school) tests positive for COVID-19, your child may need to stay home for a 2-week quarantine period. You may need to consider the feasibility of teleworking, taking leave from work, or identifying someone who can supervise your child in the event of school building closures or quarantine.	
☐ **Ask** how your school plans to help ensure that students are following practices to reduce the spread of COVID-19.	
☐ **Reinforce** the concept of physical distancing with your child.	

CHECKLIST FOR BACK TO SCHOOL

*PARENTS CAN USE THIS CHECKLIST FOR CHILDREN RETURNING BACK TO CLASSES. CDC.GOV/CORONAVIRUS

Actions to take and points to consider	Notes
☐ If your child has an Individualized Education Program (IEP) or 504 Plan or receives other learning support (e.g., tutoring), ask your school how these services will continue.	
☐ If your child receives speech, occupational or physical therapy or other related services from the school, ask your school how these services will continue.Consider packing a water bottle.	
☐ If your child receives mental health or behavioral services (e.g., social skills training, counseling), ask your school how these services will continue.	
☐ If your school uses a cohorting model, consider limiting your child's in-person out-of-school interactions to children in the same cohort or to activities where physical distancing can be maintained.	
☐ **Plan** for transportation: • If your child rides a bus, plan for your child to wear a mask on the bus and talk to your child about the importance of following bus rules and any spaced seating rules. • If carpooling, plan on every child in the carpool and the driver wearing masks for the entire trip. If your school uses the cohort model, consider finding families within your child's group/cohort at school to be part of the carpool.	

CHECKLIST FOR BACK TO SCHOOL

*PARENTS CAN USE THIS CHECKLIST FOR CHILDREN RETURNING BACK TO CLASSES. CDC.GOV/CORONAVIRUS

Actions to take and points to consider	Notes
☐ **Talk** to your school administrators and teachers about their plans for physical education and physical activity (e.g., recess). Safer options include being outdoors when possible, reducing the number of people in an indoor space, and encouraging students to stay at least 6 ft apart.	

MASKS

IS YOUR SCHOOL REQUIRING OR ENCOURAGING THE USE OF MASKS?

Actions to take and points to consider	Notes
☐ **Have** multiple masks, so you can wash them daily and have back-ups ready. Choose masks that: • Fit snugly but comfortably against the side of the face • Completely cover the nose and mouth • Are secured with ties or ear loops • Include multiple layers of fabric • Allow for breathing without restriction • Can be washed and machine dried without damage or change to shape	
☐ **Label** your child's masks clearly in a permanent marker so that they are not confused with those of other children.	

CHECKLIST FOR BACK TO SCHOOL

*PARENTS CAN USE THIS CHECKLIST FOR CHILDREN RETURNING BACK TO CLASSES, CDC.GOV/CORONAVIRUS

Actions to take and points to consider	Notes
☐ **Practice** with your child putting on and taking off masks without touching the part that covers the face.	
☐ **Explain** the importance of wearing a mask and how it protects other people from getting sick.	
☐ **Consider** talking to your child about other people who may not be able to wear masks for medical reasons (e.g., asthma).	
☐ As a family, model wearing masks, especially when you are in situations where physical distancing is difficult to maintain or impossible.	
☐ If you have a young child, help build their comfort wearing a mask and become comfortable seeing others in masks. American Academy of Pediatrics • **Praise** your child for wearing a mask correctly. • **Put a mask** on stuffed animals. Or draw a mask on a favorite book character • **Show images** of other children wearing masks. • **Allow** your child to choose their mask that meets any dress requirements your school may have.	
☐ **Consider** providing your child with a container (e.g., labeled resealable bag) to bring to school to store their mask when not wearing it (e.g., when eating).	

CHECKLIST FOR BACK TO SCHOOL

*PARENTS CAN USE THIS CHECKLIST FOR CHILDREN RETURNING BACK TO CLASSES. CDC.GOV/CORONAVIRUS

MENTAL HEALTH AND SOCIAL-EMOTIONAL WELLBEING CONSIDERATIONS

Actions to take and points to consider	Notes
☐ **Talk** with your child about how school will look different (e.g., desks far apart from each other, teachers maintaining physical distance, possibility of staying in the classroom for lunch).	
☐ **Talk** with your child about how school is going and about interactions with classmates and teachers. Find out how your child is feeling and communicate that what they may be feeling is normal.	
☐ **Anticipate** behavior changes in your child. Watch for changes like excessive crying or irritation, excessive worry or sadness, unhealthy eating or sleeping habits, difficulty concentrating, which may be signs of your child struggling with stress and anxiety.	
☐ **Try** to attend school activities and meetings. Schools may offer more of these virtually. As a parent, staying informed and connected may reduce your feelings of anxiety and provide a way for you to express any concerns you may have about your child's school.	
☐ **Ask** your school about any plans to reduce potential stigma related to having or being suspected of having COVID-19.	
☐ **Check** if your school has any systems in place to identify and provide mental health services to students in need of support. If so, identify a point of contact for these services at your school.	Name of school point person(s): Contact info:

CHECKLIST FOR BACK TO SCHOOL

*PARENTS CAN USE THIS CHECKLIST FOR CHILDREN RETURNING BACK TO CLASSES. CDC.GOV/CORONAVIRUS

Actions to take and points to consider	Notes
☐ **Check** if your school has a plan to help students adjust to being back in school. Students might need help adjusting to how COVID-19 has disrupted their daily life. Support may include school counseling and psychological services (including grief counseling), social-emotional learning (SEL)-focused programs and curricula, and peer/social support groups.	
☐ **Check** if your school will provide training for students in mindfulness, incorporating SEL into classroom curriculum (either virtually or in-person), or support a child's ability to cope with stress and anxiety. If not, consider asking about ways to add this to your child's at-home learning.	
☐ You can be a role model for your child by practicing self-care: • Take breaks • Get plenty of sleep • Exercise • Eat well • Stay socially connected	

COLOR & #BEATCOVID

SARS-CoV-2

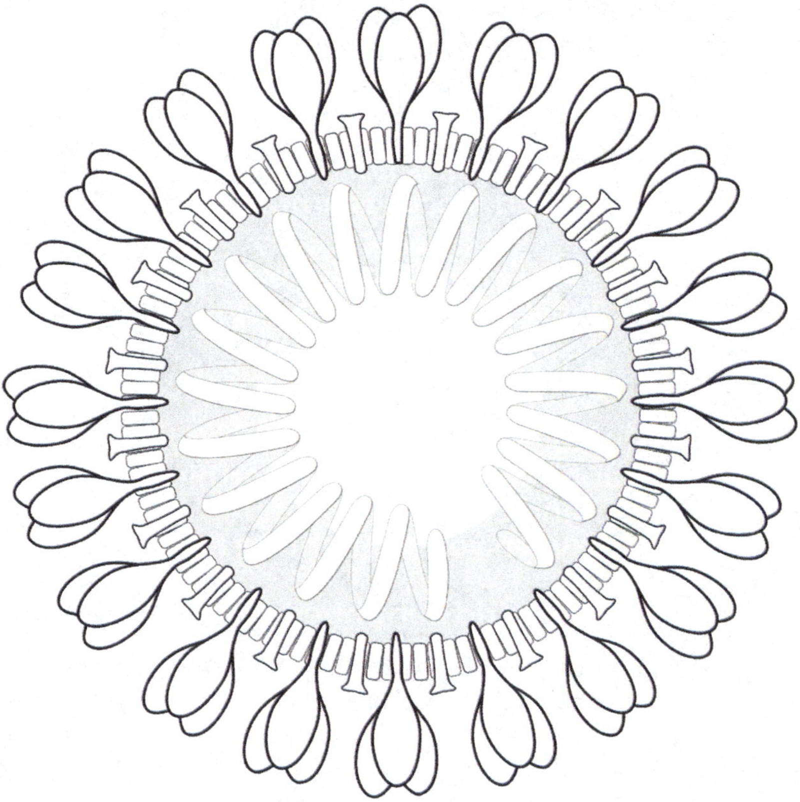

REV Med

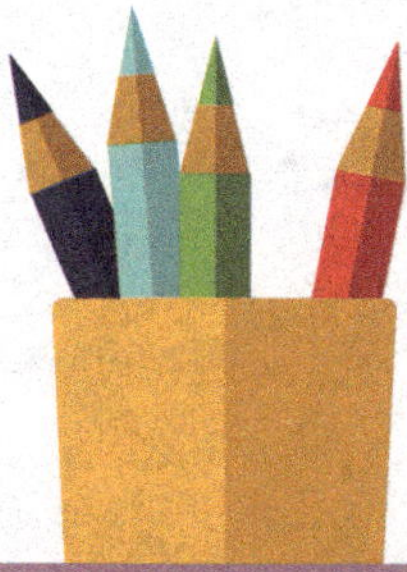

WIN A PRIZE!

Snap a picture and share your design with us on social media by using the hashtag **#BEATCOVID** and tag us **@rev.med**

www.covid19ebook.org

UPON OUR RETURN

We fell asleep in one world,
and woke up in another.

Suddenly Disney is out of magic,
Paris is no longer romantic,
New York has gone to sleep,
the Chinese wall is no longer a fortress,
and Mecca is empty.

Hugs and kisses suddenly became
weapons, and not visiting
parents and friends
became an act of love.

Suddenly, you realize that power,
beauty, and money are worthless,
and cannot get you the
oxygen you are fighting for.

The world continues its life,
and it is beautiful.
It only puts humans in cages.
I think it is sending us a message...

"You are not necessary. The air, earth,
water, and sky without you are fine.
When you come back, remember that
you are my guests. Not my masters."

LET'S ALL BE GRATEFUL

Made in the USA
Monee, IL
03 November 2026

67378305R00079